HEALTH
PROMOTION

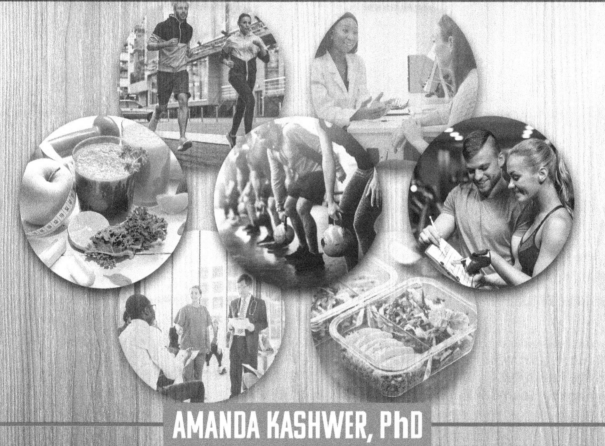

AMANDA KASHWER, PhD

Kendall Hunt
publishing company

Cover images © Shutterstock.com

Kendall Hunt
publishing company

www.kendallhunt.com
Send all inquiries to:
4050 Westmark Drive
Dubuque, IA 52004-1840

Copyright © 2019 by Kendall Hunt Publishing Company

ISBN: 978-1-5249-8856-2

Published in the United States of America

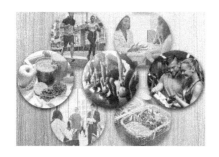

Contents

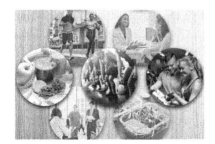

CHAPTER 1
Health Defined, Health Dimensions, and Health Determinants

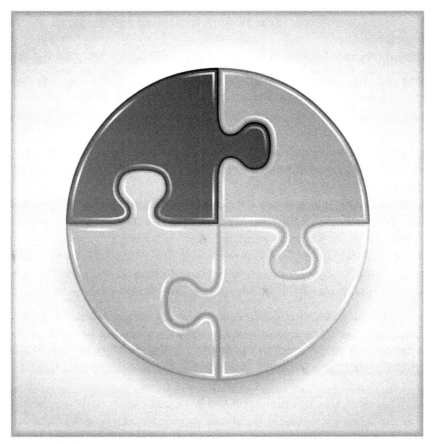

© photographer/Shutterstock.com

Health Defined

Health professionals and those preparing to be health professionals in health education and health promotion seek to understand health and to improve it for the populations and individuals that they serve. There can be no successful efforts to improve health without a clear understanding of what health is. In their efforts, health professionals will realize that people may ascribe definitions for health, illness, and disease that are not the same across populations and cultures.

For many generations, health was defined as the absence of illness and disease. Unlike the definition for health, the definitions for illness and disease may seem fairly straightforward. Illness is defined as the visible presentation of symptoms which make one feel distressed. Illness can be observed objectively by the health professional. However, for the lay person illness may mean being sick and in need of help from someone who can provide relief. The person providing relief may be a physician, folk healer, or other practitioner identified formally or informally, depending on the cultural and social orientation of the sick person.

Disease is defined as the underlying defect or malfunction within the organism. Disease may occur without illness. For an example, diabetes mellitus when it is controlled may not result in illness from diabetes. However, the individual still has diabetes. The causes of diseases and illnesses are often explored and determined as host, agent, and environmental factors. There may be differences between the practitioner and the population in determining what these factors really are. The sociocultural aspects of illness and disease present other explanations, besides carcinogens, bacteria, viruses, etc., for determining the causes or agents for illness and disease, such as "soul loss," "evil eye," demonic or spirit possession, spells, even another person for the populations that are served by health professionals.

Health is even more difficult to define than illness and disease. Examine the following definitions for health.

- Health is a state of complete physical, mental, and social well-being and not merely the absence of disease or infirmity *(World Health Organization, 1947)*.
- Health is the condition of the organism, which measures the degree to which its aggregate powers are able to function *(Oberteuffer, 1965)*.
- Health is the quality of life involving dynamic interaction and interdependence among the individual's physical well-being, his mental and emotional reactions, and the social complex in which he exists *(School Health Education Study, 1967)*.
- An integrated method of functioning which is oriented toward maximizing the potential of which the individual is capable. It requires that the individual maintain a continuum of balance and purposeful direction with the environment where he is functioning *(Dunn, 1967)*.
- Health is a state of being—a quality of life. It is something that defies definition in any precise, measurable sense. It is affected by a host of physical, mental, social, and spiritual factors which no single profession or academic discipline can effectively monitor and study *(Greene and Simons-Morton, 1990)*.

Examining these definitions, illustrates that health can be so many things, because it truly does affect so many aspects of life and is in turn affected by a great many factors. These are not likely to be the ways that the lay constituency would define health. One important factor that is observed by many health practitioners and lay persons is that health is not static, it is dynamic. The individual is always required to adapt to various factors that can impact his or her health positively or negatively. One moment an individual may be healthy, but in another instance may become ill. Health and illness cannot coexist. However, those who suffer from a disease, but who are effectively managing the disease may actually experience a high level of health.

Perhaps the following definition can best serve as a general definition that works for the professional and the populations that are served by the professionals.

> *Health is the combination of the physical, psychological, social, and spiritual dimensions of life that can be balanced in a way that produces satisfaction and joy in life.*

The definition implies that humans are not one dimensional, but multidimensional. They are not static, but dynamic, constantly impacting or being impacted by their environments. The concept of balance in these dimensions of health implies that one can compensate for the lower level of health in one dimension by improving the levels of other dimensions of health. The definition implies that the balance of these dimensions will result in satisfaction that brings a sense of fulfillment and joy that is evoked by well-being and success as the individual lives a full and healthy life. The joy that is produced is more than momentary happiness; joy is both the result of and the perpetuation of hope, faith, and love (Nobles, 2010). Healthy people are joyful people who can weather the storms and the sunshine of life's circumstances and conditions. Health, then, if viewed holistically, will impact every aspect of one's life and also be impacted by many factors in life, within the physical, social, cultural, and political environments that surround every individual. Health is not an end in itself, but the means to an end or the life goals of the individual or population.

So what exactly are these dimensions of health and what do they involve?

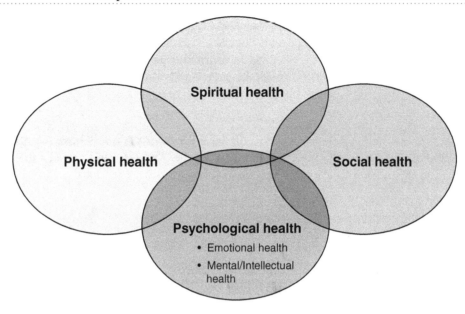

Figure 1.1. Dimensions of Health

© Kendall Hunt Publishing Company

Dimensions of Health

The origin of the word "health" is derived from the Old English word "*hale*," meaning wholeness, being whole, sound or well, strong, uninjured, of good omen—cognate with holy and implies involvement of the entire individual. Clearly this means more than the physical dimension. The nature and number of dimensions which comprise health have been debated, but health researchers and professionals are in agreement that there are varying dimensions of health and that these dimensions function in an integrated, coordinated way, never in isolation, to produce health in the individual (Dolfman, 1973). For the purposes of this text, the author presents four primary dimensions of health that can be balanced to produce joy and satisfaction:

- Physical Health
- Psychological Health (Emotional Health, Mental/Intellectual Health)
- Social Health
- Spiritual Health

Physical Health

Physical health is defined as the absence of disease and disability. It implies that the individual is functioning adequately from the perspective of physical and physiological abilities. Physical health relates to the biological integrity of the individual, incorporating the following:

- body size and shape
- sensory acuity
- susceptibility to disease
- body functioning and recuperative ability

Psychological Health

Psychological health is the appropriate intellectual, mental, and emotional practices and dimensions of the individual. Generally, psychological health reflects the following:

- values and belief systems as well as the level of self-esteem, and self-confidence
- coping skills and mechanisms
- hardiness

Within psychological health, the emotional health aspect is generally defined as the ability to feel and express the full range of human emotions, giving and receiving love, achieving a sense of fulfillment and purpose in life, and developing psychological hardiness. Mental or intellectual health encompasses the intellectual processes of reasoning, analysis, evaluation, curiosity, humor, alertness, logic, learning, and memory.

Social Health

Social health refers to the ability to perform and fulfill the expectations of our roles in society, "effectively, comfortably, with pleasure, without harming other people" (Butler, 2001). An individual's social health includes, but is not limited to the following:

- interactions and connections with others
- the ability to adapt to various social situations
- the daily behaviors and actions
- the ability to communicate effectively
- the ability to show respect
- a sense of belonging within a larger social context
- having responsibilities that often affect others and involve meeting their needs
- needs for love, intimacy, companionship, safety, and cooperation

Spiritual Health

Spiritual health has been defined by Hawks (1994) as "a high level of faith, hope, and commitment in relation to a well-defined worldview or belief system that provides a sense of meaning and purpose to existence, and that offers an ethical path to personal fulfillment which includes connectedness with self, others, and a higher power or larger reality." Banks (1980) and Butler (2001) find that the spiritual dimension of health has a unifying force within the individual that integrates all of the other dimensions of health, affecting the total health and well-being. Spiritual health may or may not be reflected in religious practices. Spiritual health is the core that makes the following possible:

- the ability to discover, articulate, and act on one's basic purpose in life,
- learning how to give and receive love, joy, and peace,
- contributing to the improvement of the spiritual health of others,
- pursuing a fulfilling and meaningful life,
- transcending the self with a sense of selflessness, or empathy, for others and establishing a commitment to a power beyond the natural and rational,
- having the power to pursue successes in life through a defined set of moral principles and ethics.

Some research indicates that the spiritual component may actually provide the unifying context for all other components of health.

Other Health-Related Definitions

Wellness

While the terms "health" and "wellness" are often used interchangeably, they are not synonyms (Penhollow, 2012). Wellness is a concept that describes the process of adopting behaviors that determine one's quality of life. Anspaugh et al., (1997) pronounced that wellness means engaging in attitudes and behaviors that enhance the quality of life and maximize personal potential. The dimensions of wellness are very similar to those in the description of health, but may also include the dimensions of environmental, and occupational wellness. Often health professionals refer to the wellness scale that indicates the quality of life as a range from optimal wellness to premature death. The individual can choose to exercise control over a variety of life factors that will influence the level or ranking of wellness. The more positive life factors present in a person's life at any given time, the greater is the likelihood of optimal health and wellness. If one approaches wellness as a continuum with the midpoint as no signs or symptoms of disease, as in Figure 1.2, one's choices in behaviors can move

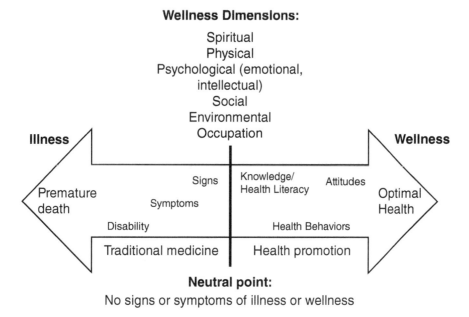

Figure 1.2. A Continuum for Wellness

© Kendall Hunt Publishing Company

the individual toward illness or premature death or the individual may choose behaviors that move him/her toward wellness and optimal health.

Personal Health

Personal health is the actions and decisions made by the individual that affect his or her own health. It is important to note that some of the decisions and actions may be impacted by factors outside of the person's control.

Community Health and Population Health

People interact with each other in many ways for many reasons. These interactions with common bonds are generally referred to as community. Community is defined as a unified body of people with common interests living in a particular area; an interacting population of various kinds of individuals in a common location; or, a "body of persons with a common history, ethnic heritage, political interests, or social and economic characteristics (Merriam-Webster Dictionary, 2013). Community health refers to the health status, issues, activities, and events of a community. This includes the organized responsibilities of public health, school health, transportation safety, other tax-supported functions, with voluntary and private actions, to promote and protect the health of local populations identified as communities. Sometimes the term population health is used. Population health refers to the health status and the conditions influencing the health of a category of people (for example, women, adolescents, prisoners) whether or not the people included in the category define themselves as a community.

Determinants of Health

An examination of the health of individuals and communities will lead to determining how certain health, illness, and disease conditions come into existence. Throughout history, societies have sought answers to the questions about how to achieve greater health and avoid injury, disease, illness, and premature death. There are various models and theories on disease and disease interventions to reduce the transmission of diseases and to promote health. The following have helped health professionals to arrive at the most current understandings about what factors determine health and enable health care providers to help individuals and communities reach greater health and quality of their lives.

Communicable disease is a disease that requires a pathogen to spread the disease. The communicable disease model describes the spread of disease requiring the elements of an agent, host, and environment. Figure 1.3 illustrates the traditional epidemiologic triad model for the transmission of infectious disease resulting from the interaction among the host, the agent, and the environment. Figure 1.4 shows the transmission occurring as the agent moves from the host or reservoir through a portal of exit by a mode of transmission and then enters through a portal of entry to infect a new host. This disease process is referred to as the chain of infection and will continue until the chain is broken.

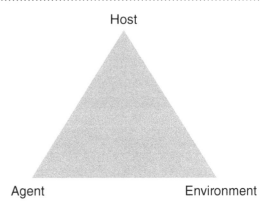

Figure 1.3.   Communicable Disease Model

These models do help the health professionals working in health education and health promotion explain and intervene in reducing the spread of communicable or infectious disease. In more recent years, there is greater knowledge and experience related to diseases that are communicable and those that are the result of lifestyle choices. Canada in the 1970's implemented a national plan to insure health care for all Canadians. Canadian health professionals began to examine the health field rather than the health care system to broaden their assessment of the many matters that impact and affect the health of their people. The Lalonde Report, *A New Perspective on the Health of Canadians* (1974), introduced the concept of the "health field" which at that time consisted of four categories of elements that could influence death and disease for humans: human biology or heredity, environment, lifestyle or behavior, and inadequacies of the health care services. Shortly after the Lalonde Report the United States government officially entered health promotion with the publication of *Healthy People: The Surgeon General's Report on Health Promotion and Disease Prevention* (1979). No longer was the focus totally on the treatment of disease, but the emphasis moved to the prevention of illness and health promotion.

For many years, the Health Field Concept provided a framework that is used by many health professionals to identify causes of morbidity and mortality, by examining the contributions of heredity, environment, health care services, and behavior to a variety of health conditions and problems. In the most recent years, the Health Field Concept has yielded to the use of the term "determinants of health," as a way to assess and explain the many factors that determine the health of populations. According to McGinnis, et al., (2001), the impacts of these determinants on premature mortality are distributed as ". . . genetic predispositions, about 30%, social circumstances, 15%, environmental exposures, 5%, behavioral patterns, 40%; and shortfalls in medical care about 10%." It is important to note that while these determinants are listed individually, they do interact and interconnect having impacts on each other and reflecting the total health of the individual, the family, and the community.

According to the 2011 Joint Committee on Health Education and Health Promotion Terminology (2012), determinants of health are "the range of personal, social, economic, and environmental factors that influence health status." The categories of determinants affecting individual and community levels of health are:

- Genetic Factors/Heredity (Micro/Internal Environment)
- Physical Environment
- Social Environment
- Health Care
- Personal Health Behavior And Lifestyle Choices

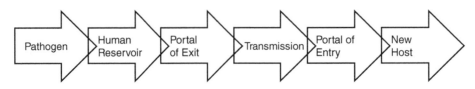

Figure 1.4.   Chain of Infection Model

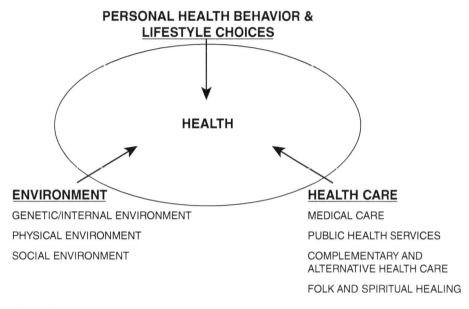

Figure 1.5.   Categories of the Determinants of Health

Genetic Factors/Heredity

Generally, it is believed that there are a number of factors affecting our health over which we have little control. However, it may be difficult to separate the influences of heredity from those of culture and social circumstances for individuals and groups of people. The genetic factors determining the health of individuals and populations include the following:

- Genetic traits affecting optimal functioning
- Sex
- Body size and composition

The Physical Environment

The physical environment has great importance and influence on the health of individuals and communities. Increasingly, individuals, communities, and health professionals understand how pollution and contamination of the water, air, and food supply are linked to greater incidence and prevalence of a variety of diseases and allergic reactions. Some of the determinants of health in the physical environment are:

- Air
- Water
- Soil
- Animal life
- Plant life
- Natural disasters

The Social Environment

Social scientists and social epidemiologists examine the relationships of health problems and social factors. They try to determine the influence on health and their associations with health. Research has documented the importance of social variables in predicting and describing health and health problems. John Ratcliffe (1980) believed that society's social structure greatly affects the lives and the health of all people.

In many communities, socially designed systems have become more important than the physical environment to individual survival, because they control the distribution of and access to those very factors that determine mortality and morbidity levels. To be sure, the physical environment still exacts a great toll through incidents such as hurricanes, tornadoes, earthquakes, tidal waves, floods, etc. Nevertheless, the socioeconomic systems created by and for people constitute, to all intents and purposes, the human individual's "natural" environment (Ratcliffe, 1980). Some of the following factors can determine the health and quality of life for individuals and populations.

- Culture
- Socioeconomic factors
  - Social class
  - Personal income
  - Economy
  - Residence
- Politics
- Race and ethnicity
- Education
- Gender
- Religion
- Resources
- Community & societal organization
- Population density
- Crowding
- The pace of modern civilization
- Stressful life events
- War
- The health care environment

Health Care

Access to quality medical care and public health services can help individuals and populations experience better health. However, health care professionals must always be conscious that diverse populations may also participate in complementary and alternative health care, as well as folk healing and spiritual healing experiences. The determinants of health care will include the following:

- Medical care
- Public health services
- Complementary and alternative health care
- Folk and spiritual healing

Personal Health Behaviors and Lifestyle Choices

Most advances in optimal health and wellness in the United States have not resulted from advances in medical care, but from many of the environmental improvements and public health advances. Evidence demonstrates that the most important factors in improving health in modern societies have been improved nutrition, well-nourished babies, children, and adolescents, and relative affluence. The individual can make lifestyle changes that affect health positively or negatively, in spite of the social environment. It is in this category of determinants that health educators focus great effort. Behavior changes have great impact on health and the quality of one's life. The leading causes of death in the United States are cancers and cardiovascular diseases, which are strongly linked to lifestyle and behaviors. The following factors are supported by much research and have greatly impacted on improved health.

- Nutritional and dietary behaviors and status
- Physical activity and exercise patterns
- Adequate sleep
- Maintaining appropriate weight

- Avoidance of inappropriate use of alcohol and illegal drugs
- No tobacco use
- Prevention of unintentional injuries
- Appropriate management of stress
- Use of preventive health services

Just as there are behaviors that support optimal health there are also behaviors that cause health problems (Kolbe, 1993).

- Drug and alcohol abuse
- Risky behaviors that result in unintentional and intentional injuries
- Sexual behaviors that result in unwanted pregnancy and sexually transmitted diseases, including HIV infection
- Tobacco use
- Excessive consumption of fat and calories
- Insufficient physical activity

Risk Factors

The Health Field Concept and the Determinants of Health provide those who research and practice health education and health promotion with a framework to study and intervene with health. Such a framework helps health professionals to target factors that generate or influence the health and quality of life for the individuals, groups, and communities served. The study of determinants of health assists health professionals to target risks that are associated with disease or poor health outcomes. Risk factors are defined by the World Health the Organization as ". . . any attribute, characteristic or exposure of an individual that increases the likelihood of developing a disease or injury. Some examples of the more important risk factors are underweight, morbid obesity, unsafe sex, high blood pressure, tobacco and alcohol consumption, and unsafe water, sanitation and hygiene (2013)." A risk factor increases the probability of developing disease, disability, injury, or premature death, but does not guarantee that those with the risk factor will suffer poor health outcomes. Risk factors may be categorized as modifiable risk factors (changeable or controllable) or nonmodifiable risk factors (nonchangeable or noncontrollable). Modifiable risk factors may include smoking behaviors, sedentary lifestyle, poor nutritional habits, and poor dental care. Nonmodifiable risk factors are inherited genetic factors, race, age, sex: things that cannot be changed by the individual. Professionals involved in health education and health promotion have major responsibility for helping clients identify and control risk factors that are modifiable (Cottrell et al., 2012).

References

Anspaugh, D. J., and G. Ezell. 1995. *Teaching Today's Health,* 4th ed. Boston: Allyn & Bacon.

Butler, J. Thomas. 2001. *Principles of Health Education & Health Promotion,* 3rd ed. Belmont, CA: Wadsworth/ Thomason Learning.

Cottrell, R. R., J. T. Girvan, and J. F. McKenzie. 2012. *Principles and Foundations of Health Promotion and Education.* Boston: Benjamin Cummings.

Dolfman, M. L. 1973. "The Concept of Health: An Historic and Analytic Examination." *Journal of School Health* 43 (8): 491–7.

Dunn, H. 1967. *High Level Wellness.* Arlington, VA: R. W. Beatty.

Hawks, S. 1994. "Spiritual Health: Definition and Theory." *Wellness Perspectives: Research, Theory and Practice* 10 (4): 3–13.

Joint Committee on Health Education and Promotion Terminology. 2012. "Report of the 2011 Joint Committee on Health Education and Promotion Terminology." *American Journal of Health Education* 43 (2).

Kolbe, L. J. 1993. "Developing a Plan of Action to Institutionalize Comprehensive School Health Education Programs in the United States." *Journal of School Health* 63 (1): 12–13.

Laframboise, H. L. 1973. "Health Policy: Breaking It Down into Manageable Segments." *Journal of the Canadian Medical Association, 108* (February 3). 388–393.

Lalonde, M. 1974. *A New Perspective on the Health of Canadians: A Working Document.* Ottawa, Canada: Ministry of National Health and Welfare.

McGinnis, J. M., and W. H. Foege. 1993. "Actual Causes of Death in the United States." *Journal of the American Medical Association* 2 (18): 2207–12.

McGinnis, J. M., W. H. Williams-Russo, and J. R. Knickman. 2002. "The Case for More Active Policy Attention to Health Promotion." *Health Affairs* 21 (2): 78–93.

Nobles, Sherman. 2010. "Joy is Not Happiness?" *Theologia.* Retrieved May 18, 2013, from http://theologica. ning.com/profiles/blogs/joy-is-not-happiness.

Oberteuffer, D. 1960. *School Health Education: A Textbook for Teachers, Nurses, and Other Professional Personnel.* New York: Harper and Brothers.

Penhollow, T. M. 2012. *Points to Health: Theory and Practice of Health Education and Health Behavior.* Dubuque, IA: Kendall Hunt Publishing Company.

Simons-Morton, B. G., W. H. Greene, and N. Gottlieb. 1995. *Introduction to Health Education and Health Promotion.* Long Grove, IL: Waveland Press, Inc.

Sliepcevich, E. M. 1967. "Health Education: A Conceptual Approach to Curriculum Design." In E. M. Sliepcevich. *School Health Education Study.* St Paul: 3M Education Press.

World Health Organization. 1947. Preamble to the Constitution of the World Health Organization as adopted by the International Health Conference, New York, 19–22 June 1946; signed on 22 July 1946 by the representatives of 61 States (Official Records of the World Health Organization, no. 2, p. 100) and entered into force on 7 April 1948.

World Health Organization. 2013. http://www.who.int/topics/risk_factors/en/. Retrieved May 25, 2013.

Application Opportunity

Now that you have studied the definitions for health, its dimensions, and its determinants, return to your definition for health that you wrote in the prologue.

1. Is your definition, written in the prologue, the same as the definition(s) you studied in chapter 1?

2. What are the similarities?

3. What are the differences?

4. Which definition would serve you best as a health professional? Why?

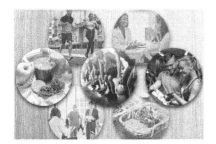

CHAPTER 2
Health Behavior, Health Education, and Health Promotion

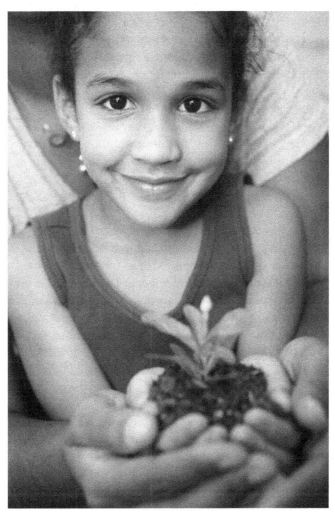

© photographer/Shutterstock.com

Health Behavior

While heredity, environment, and medical care have profound influences on the health and quality of life that every individual experiences, health behavior, or lifestyle is the greatest determinant that impacts morbidity and premature death. Poor health behaviors account for as much as 40% of the morbidity and premature death in the United States' population (McGinnis et al., 2002). Lifestyle reflects practices and behavioral patterns in the individual and population that are influenced by one's cultural heritage, social relationships, social and economic circumstances, geography, and personality. While all of these factors do influence behaviors, the individual makes many decisions on his or her own, which, in turn, impact the person's health and the quality of life. Individuals can make the decision to adopt behaviors that are health enhancing or disease producing. The individual can choose to improve the level of physical activity, avoid the use of tobacco, improve the intakes of fruits and vegetables, or avoid risky sexual behavior. The foundational basis for health education and health promotion is that individuals can voluntarily make personal choices to experience the best health outcomes. It is incumbent on the health education specialists to know the factors that influence the behaviors and lifestyle choices of the individuals and target populations that they serve. Such knowledge and experience will assist the health education specialist in facilitating changed health behaviors in the target population and in individuals.

David Gochman (1982, 1997) defines health behavior as "those personal attributes such as beliefs, expectations, motive, values, perceptions and other cognitive elements; personality characteristics, including affective and emotional states and traits; and behavioral patterns, actions and habits that relate to health maintenance, health restoration, and health improvement." This definition underscores three foci for health education specialists in helping to enhance health behaviors in individuals, groups and communities: health maintenance, health restoration, and the improvement of health.

The greatest challenge to specialists in health education and health promotion is to help individuals make the best choices for health. People will make poor choices if they do not relate health to their personal life goals, if they do not value health, if they like risk-taking, and if they are unaware of the risks for sickness or death connected to their behaviors. People will make poor choices if they lack the knowledge and the skills necessary to change their behaviors to support optimal health.

There are three categories of factors that influence all of the health choices that people make. They are predisposing factors, enabling factors, and reinforcing factors.

Predisposing factors are the antecedents of a behavior; they are the things that the individual brings to the point of making a decision or choice. These factors include demographic variables such as age, sex, gender, education, race, ethnicity, and socioeconomic conditions. Predisposing factors also consist of life experiences, values, beliefs, cultural perspectives, attitudes, and knowledge. The knowledge and attitudes may be accurate or erroneous. The health education specialists must determine what the person brings to the decision making process. This is an important key to the health education and health promotion process.

The second category of factors that influence all behaviors is enabling factors. Enabling factors are also present before the behavior occurs. Enabling factors are the person's arsenal of skills and abilities that they bring to their decisions related to behavior. Enabling factors will include the availability of health resources, affordable health care and services, or the easy availability of those things that may negatively affect health choices as well.

Reinforcing factors are the third category of factors which occur after the behavior. These are the things that can encourage the repetition of a new behavior or the extinguishing of the behavior. Reinforcing factors may include support of family and friends, feedback, and reward from instructors or employers. Often the good feelings that one experiences from improving health by a positive behavior change may help the individual to repeat the behavior, allowing the behavior to become a positive health habit.

Health Education

According to the Joint Committee on Health Education and Health Promotion Terminology (2012), health education is "Any combination of planned learning experiences using evidence based practices and/or sound theories that provide the opportunity to acquire knowledge, attitudes, and skills needed to adopt and maintain healthy behaviors." Health education is also described as a planned process that combines various educational experiences to facilitate voluntary adaptations or establishment of behaviors that are conducive to health (Green and Kreuter, 1999). The practice of health education focuses on a goal of helping people (individuals, families, groups, and communities) choose a pattern of behaviors which moves them toward optimal health rather than the reverse and to give them the ability to avoid many of the imbalances, diseases, and accidents of life (Oberteuffer et al., 1972). Even though the field of health education has many practitioners, this goal generally describes the mission of the field and its professionals.

The fundamental principle of health education is that individuals, families, and communities can be taught to assume responsibility for their own health and, to some extent, for the health of others. The facilitation of voluntary individual and community behavior change without violating individual freedoms guaranteed by the United States Constitution is the challenge for health education professionals.

In order to bring about the voluntary changes in these persons for behaviors that support health, there is the process of health education. Butler (2001) describes the process of health education as going beyond the memorization of information, but must also include the following:

1. The process begins with a planned intervention based on a health issue, with stated goals, objectives, activities, and evaluation criteria.
2. The intervention occurs in a specified setting and at a specified time.
3. The components of a health education intervention or program are the sequential introduction of health concepts at appropriate learning levels at each stage of the learning process and resulting in changed behaviors to support optimal health.
4. The planned intervention comprehensively helps the learner to realize how various aspects of health are interrelated and how all health behavior affects the quality of life.
5. The learner interacts with a qualified and competent educator.

In most cases the health education process improves the health knowledge base, but more importantly, there will be enriched attitudes to support behavior change, enhanced skill development, values awareness that can advance decision-making in the individual, family, and community, leading to improved health and quality of life. Positive outcomes will depend on how effectively the health education specialist plans the process.

Common misconceptions about health education are that anyone can teach health, that anyone can write an effective health education curriculum, and that health education is hygiene class. It is important to note that improving the quality of life and health status of individuals, groups, and communities are very complex and not changed in short periods of time. In examining the process for health education, the health educators must be competent in program planning, implementation, program evaluation, and in quality service delivery. Health education interventions require the health education specialist to be professionally prepared to perform various roles depending on the nature and needs of the learners. Most health education interventions will center on teaching, training counseling and consulting (Simons-Morton et al., 1995).

Teaching

The health education specialist employs a variety of strategies, methods, and activities to help individuals, groups, and communities establish and change patterns of behavior to improve health. The health education specialist's success is dependent on what to teach and how to teach it. Conveying information alone is not sufficient to effect behavior change, because knowledge does not necessarily change attitudes or behavior.

Training

The health education specialist teaches other health professionals and volunteers how to accomplish health education goals and objectives and how to employ health education methods.

Counseling

In counseling, the health education specialist is involved in an interpersonal process of guidance that helps people learn how to achieve personal growth, improve interpersonal growth and relationships, resolve problems, make decisions, and change behavior for optimal health.

Consulting

The health education specialist employs the process by which his/her knowledge and experience are used to help another professional or organization make better decisions or cope with problems more effectively to address a group or population's health status.

The discipline and practice of health education are supported by contributions from a vast body of research in the health sciences and the social sciences that can help to reduce the risks for poor health through behavior change. The primary contributors are public health, behavioral sciences, and education. Public health contributes health statistics for epidemiologic data as the health education specialist assesses the health status of target populations. Public health also contributes to the understanding of health issues in the environment, personal lifestyles, medical care, population dynamics, biomedical science, and epidemiology. Behavioral sciences are the integration of knowledge from psychology, sociology, and cultural anthropology, providing a foundation for understanding human health behaviors. The behavioral sciences contribute greatly to defining the determinants of behavior that are key to healthful behavior change, which is the desired outcome for health education practice. Education is the study of teaching and learning which is central to health education. Education provides the health education specialist with learning theory, educational psychology, human development, curriculum development, and pedagogy. Measurement and testing are also contributions from education (Butler, 2001).

Health education has transitioned from its earliest appearance as a profession. Health education specialists are now central to the health promotion efforts that many local, state and national organizations are engaged in as these agencies seek to address the many health challenges facing the nation and the world. Sometimes the terms of health education and health promotion are used interchangeably; however, health education has the longest history regarding its extensive mission within society and health care (Penhollow, 2012).

Health Promotion

The Joint Committee on Health Education and Promotion Terminology (2012) defines health promotion as "any planned combination of educational, political, environmental, regulatory, or organizational mechanisms that support actions and conditions of living conducive to the health of individuals, groups and communities." O'Donnell (2009) defines health promotion as both art and science combined to help people ". . . discover the synergies between their core passions and optimal health, enhancing their motivation to strive for optimal health, and supporting them in changing their lifestyle to move toward a state of optimal health." He additionally emphasized the important and dynamic balance among physical, emotional, social, spiritual, and intellectual health. The role of health education in health promotion can be observed in lifestyle changes that are facilitated through selected combinations of learning experiences and strategies. Health promotion efforts also seek to enhance awareness, encourage commitment to action, and build needed skills. According to O'Donnell (2009), health promotion's most important contribution is "through the creation of opportunities that open access to environments that make positive health practices the easiest choice."

Health promotion is a broad field encompassing educational, social, economic, and political efforts to improve the health of a population, emerging as an unifying concept bringing a number of separate fields under one umbrella. Health promotion enables people to take control and responsibility for their health, requires close cooperation of heterogeneous sectors, and combines diverse methods or approaches, while encouraging effective and concrete public participation. Many of the strategies in health promotion come from an ecological perspective that seeks to empower individuals, groups, communities in developing behaviors and lifestyles that enhance health.

Health promotion is made up of three important areas of practice, each of which has a vital role in achieving health for the individual and the community: health education, health protection, and disease prevention. These are commonly referred to as the triad of health promotion. The professionals in these areas of practice work together providing the best opportunities for individuals, groups, and communities to make choices for optimal health.

Health Education

Health education is at the core of total health promotion programming. Health education professionals provide knowledge, skill development, and support that help clients understand their options and voluntarily choose health behaviors for optimal health and high quality of life. While other professions are involved in the work of health promotion, health education is the primary profession devoted to health promotion and whose practitioners are trained in a range of health promotion processes (Simons-Morton, Greens, & Gottlieb, 1995). Health education is a planned process which usually combines educational experiences to facilitate voluntary adaptations or establishment of behavior conducive to health. Health education specialists educate individuals about their own health as well as educate the media, elected officials, and community leaders.

Disease Prevention

Disease prevention is a major emphasis for health promotion. Disease prevention, according to the Joint Committee (2012), "is the process of reducing risks and alleviating disease to promote, preserve, and restore health and minimize suffering and distress." Prevention consists of three levels of prevention. Each has specific implications for the health education specialist or health promoter. Each requires different objectives, methods, and interventions (programs).

Primary prevention emphasizes interventions to avert disease, illness, injury, or deterioration of health before these occur. Primary prevention may include vaccinations and immunizations for children and adults. Vaccinations will cause the production of antibodies which will prevent future cases of a disease so that people will not get sick.

Another example of primary prevention is early pregnancy interventions that teach pregnant women to adopt healthy behaviors that support healthy pregnancies, deliveries, and healthy newborns. There are legislative actions that are considered primary prevention, such as water fluoridation, seat belt laws, laws requiring child restraint seats in vehicles, laws requiring immunizations before attending school, and laws requiring food handlers to be periodically tested for infectious diseases. All of these actions are designed to prevent diseases, disabilities, and injuries. It is at the primary prevention level that health education specialists and health promoters can have their greatest impact on the health of a population. Primary prevention is the most cost-effective form of disease prevention.

Secondary prevention identifies diseases at their earliest stages and applies appropriate measures to limit the consequences and severity of the disease. The efforts in secondary prevention center on early detection and treatment of diseases. The focus is curative and this has been the primary focus for medicine. Secondary prevention directs resources to identify diseases at the earliest stage possible so that the damage from the disease can be limited. Examples of secondary prevention are mammograms, Pap tests, testicular exams, regular blood pressure measurements, measurements for blood cholesterol and blood glucose, and vision examinations. The health education specialist or patient educator in many of these situations plays an important role in getting clients to schedule tests for early detection of diseases and for providing the knowledge and skills for clients to reduce or avoid the destructive disease progress and improve their health.

Tertiary prevention helps people who already have diseases and disabilities. Tertiary prevention prescribes specific interventions to limit the effects of disabilities and diseases and may also prevent the recurrence of disease. The level of tertiary prevention will depend on the medical care that is available to the individual or community. Some of the critical components of tertiary care are rehabilitation services, physical therapy, and occupational therapy that may not be available to individuals because of costs or lack of health insurance, or because such services are not available in some communities. This level of tertiary prevention will depend heavily on surgery, medications, and counseling. Tertiary prevention and the care required at this level is the most expensive, when compared to secondary or primary prevention. It is the least cost-effective in preventing illness and disease.

Health Protection

Health protection includes ". . . the legal or fiscal controls, other regulations and policies, and voluntary codes of practice, aimed at the enhancement of positive health and the prevention of ill health" (Downie et al., 1996). Health education specialists and promoters must overcome many barriers to health protection. The mission of health protection is to provide legislative, political, and social constructs that reduce the likelihood of people behaving in unsafe ways or to remove environmental hazards that impact health outcomes. Rules that forbid smoking in the workplace, laws that tax tobacco products, and regulations forbidding smoking in schools and other public places are all examples of health protections that have reduced smoking among some populations and reduced the likelihood that these populations will develop certain cancers or cardiovascular diseases. Many efforts to establish and enforce health protection have met with great opposition because it violates one of the tenets of health education and health promotion: individuals have the constitutional right to voluntarily choose to change behaviors that promote health. This opposition to certain efforts for health protection is found among lobbying organizations, political groups, and industries, with just as many groups and organizations supporting these efforts.

The Triad of Health Promotion

Tannahill (1985) noted that these three areas that make up health promotion generate seven domains. As the health professionals in disease prevention, health education, and health protection relate to, intersect, and interact with each other, the following seven domains arise in health promotion.

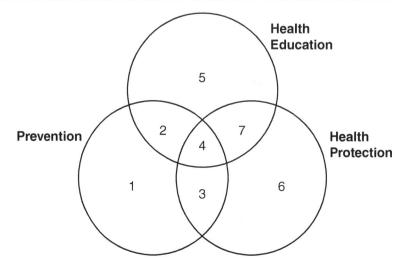

Figure 2.1. The seven domains produced by triad of health promotion

Tannahill, A. (1985). "What is health promotion?" *Health Education Journal*, 44, 167–8.

1. Prevention:
   This domain includes the primary, secondary, and tertiary prevention measures and programs.
2. Lifestyle:
   This domain results from the interaction of disease prevention and health education. It is comprised of educational efforts to influence lifestyle to prevent health problems and to encourage participation in preventive services.
3. Preventive Policies:
   This domain results from the interaction of disease prevention and health protection. This domain represents preventive health protection. Examples of the work in this domain would be water purification, water fluoridation, restaurant inspections, etc. The domain would be considered to be policy commitments to preventive efforts under domain 1.
4. Policy Maker Education:
   The interactions among disease prevention, health education, and health protection gives rise to professionals and services that are involved in preparing and stimulating the social environment, legislators, and policy makers to support preventive health protection actions and measures.
5. Health Education:
   This domain involves all aspects of health education that influences health behaviors for positive health outcomes.
6. Health Protection:
   This domain supports the implementation of policies and the commitment of funds for health protection efforts.
7. Policy Support:
   This domain is an interaction of health education and health protection. It involves a policy commitment to positive health and raising awareness and securing support for positive health protection measures among the public and policy makers.

Primary Themes in Health Promotion

Health promotion seeks improved health and quality of life for the individual, but also for groups and the general population. In observing the many health promotion interventions and strategies, it becomes obvious that there are specific themes in health promotion efforts. Some of these themes are listed below (Butler, 2001).

- Empowerment:
  Empowerment is a multilevel construct that involves people assuming control over their lives in the context of their social and political environment.

■ Ecological Perspective:
The ecological perspective views health as a product of the interdependence of the individual and subsystems of the ecosystem such as family, culture, and physical and social environment.

■ Community Organization:
Community organization is a multi-phased process by which community groups are helped to produce change and develop their community for improved health and quality of life.

■ Individual Behavior:
Although we emphasize social and economic factors, we must not forget the crucial role of individual behavior in one's health.

■ Official Recognition:
Many official United States, Canadian, and international pronouncements have recognized the importance of health promotion and have laid a groundwork for its continued growth.

References

Butler, J. T. 2001. *Principles of Health Education and Health Promotion,* 3rd ed. Belmont, CA: Wadsworth/ Thomson Learning.

Downie, R. S., C. Tannahill, and A. Tannahill. 1996. *Health Promotion: Models and Values,* 2nd ed. Oxford, England: Oxford University Press.

Doyle, E., and S. Ward. 2005. *The Process of Community Health Education and Promotion.* Long Grove, IL: Waveland Press, Inc.

Gochman, D. S. 1982. "Labels, Systems, and Motives: Some Perspectives on Future Research." *Health Education Quarterly* 9: 167–74.

Gochman, D. S. 1997. "Health Behavior Research: Definitions and Diversity." In D. S. Gochman (Ed.), *Handbook of Health Behavior Research: Vol.1. Personal and Social Determinants.* New York: Plenum Press.

Green, L. W., and M. W. Kreuter. 1999. *Health Promotion Planning: An Educational and Ecological Approach,* 3rd ed. Mountain View, CA: Mayfield.

Joint Committee on Health Education and Promotion Terminology. 2012. "Report of the 2011 Joint Committee on Health Education and Promotion Terminology." *American Journal of Health Education* 43 (2).

McGinnis, J. M., P. Williams-Russo, and J. R. Knickman. 2002. "The case for more active policy attention to health promotion." *Health Affairs* 21 (2): 78–93.

Oberteuffer, D., O. A. Harrelson, and M. B. Pollock. 1972. *School Health Education,* 5th ed. New York: Harper & Row.

O'Donnell Michael P. 2009. "Definition of Health Promotion 2.0: Embracing Passion, Enhancing Motivation, Recognizing Dynamic Balance, and Creating Opportunities." *American Journal of Health Promotion: September/October 2009* 24 (1): iv.

Penhollow, T. M. 2012. *Points to Health: Theory and Practice of Health Education and Health Behavior.* Dubuque, IA: Kendall Hunt Publishing Company.

Simons-Morton, B. G., W. H. Greens, and N. H. Gottlieb. 1995. *Introduction to Health Education and Health Promotion,* 2nd ed. Prospects Heights, IL: Waveland.

Tannahill, A. 1985. What is Health Promotion? *Health Education Journal* 44: 167–8.

Application Opportunity

Activity A

As you read about health behavior, health education, and health promotion, what in these fields or areas appeal to you and relates to your future preparation for a career in the health care field? Why?

Activity B

Examine the themes of health promotion. As a future health professional, which of the primary themes in health promotion speaks to your passion about helping people improve the quality of their lives? Why?

Activity C

As you read this chapter and answered the questions in Activities A and B, you may have realized that to perform as a health professional in health education and health promotion, your personal life's philosophy is important and foundational. Write below your philosophical foundation that you would bring to health education and health promotion.

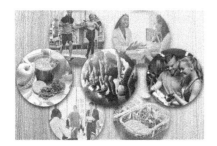

CHAPTER 3
History of Health Education

The concept of educating about health has been around since ancient times; however, the history of health education and health promotion as an emerging profession is just over 100 years old. Learning about the history of health education allows for an appreciation of the struggles and obstacles faced by pioneers of the profession. One cannot fully appreciate the present condition of the profession without first knowing about its origin. This allows health professionals and others of interest to learn from the past and observe the progress and trends made over time. This chapter provides a historical account of health education and health promotion from the earliest human records to the present condition of public health in the United States. The chapter mainly focuses on Europe and Northern Africa, as these areas had the greatest influence on the nation's history of medicine and health care.

Timeline by Era

Early Humans

The earliest humans fundamentally learned health-related knowledge and discovered medicines through observation, trial, and error. In those days, **morbidity** (disease) and **mortality** (death) were much more common than health and longevity. Early civilizations were largely puzzled by disease and death. In an attempt to make sense of these events, they believed in the influence of magic, evil spirits, and gods. To prevent the spread of disease, early humans made sacrifices to the gods, rituals of the time were observed, and haunted places were avoided. Amulets and charms were worn by early civilizations, and spells and chants were performed as a way to help protect people from disease (Duncan, 1988).

Medical lore of the past from the earliest humans was handed down from generation to generation. Evidence of the earliest efforts at public and community health can be discovered in Northern India. Excavations dating from around 2000 B.C. have evidence of bathrooms, drains, and covered sewers. The oldest known written health-related documents are the Code of Hammurabi (2080 B.C.) and the Smith Papyri (1600 B.C.) (Cottrell, Girvan, & McKenzie, 2012). The **Code of Hammurabi**, named after the king of Babylon, was the earliest written record concerning public health which included laws pertaining to health care practices and physician fees. The **Smith Papyri** described various surgical techniques of the time.

Egyptians (3000–1500 B.C.)

In virtually every culture containing documented historical accounts, people turned to some type of physician or medicine man for health-related information (education, treatment, and cures) (Green & Simons-Morton, 1990). In Egypt, as well as in a number of other cultures, this role was held by the priests. The Egyptians made significant progress in the area of public health. The Egyptians were known for their cleanliness and considered to be the healthiest of ancient civilizations. They constructed earth privies for sewage, as well as public draining pipes. The Egyptian people knew over 700 different drugs and exercised a number of pharmacological remedies, such as using the fat of a serpent, mammalian entrails, tissues, and organs (Pickett & Hanlon, 1990). Spells, incantations, exorcisms, prescriptions, and clinical observations were also performed during this time period (Libby, 1922).

Hebrews (1500 B.C.)

The Hebrews extended Egyptian hygienic thought and medicinal practices. Hebrews relied on strict codes which controlled virtually all behavior. The assignment of the Sabbath as a day of rest, which is still observed by Orthodox Jews today, matches the severe restriction of activities on the seventh day of the week-Sunday. The king engaged in no official business and physicians were not permitted to treat the sick on the day of the Sabbath (Health Guidance, 2011).

The Hebrews were responsible for the first written hygienic code, the **Book of Leviticus**. The Book of Leviticus contained information on the following:

- Cleanliness of the body
- Protecting against contagious diseases
- Isolation for lepers
- Disinfection of dwellings after an illness
- Disposal of excreta and refuse
- Sanitation of campsites
- Protection of food and water supplies
- Hygiene of maternity

Greeks (1000–400 B.C.)

The history of health care in the Greek culture is fascinating. The Greeks took information from the Babylonians, Egyptians, Hebrews and other people of the eastern Mediterranean. In early Greek culture, the priesthood played a large role in the public health of the community. The Greeks were the first people to place emphasis on the prevention of disease rather than the treatment of disease. They emphasized balance among the physical (athletics), mental (philosophy), and spiritual (theology) (Cottrell et al., 2012). The Greeks were active in the practice of community sanitation and supplemented water from city wells by water from the mountains if necessary.

> According to Greek mythology, **Asclepius**, the son of Apollo and a Thessalian chief who had received instruction in the use of drugs, was endowed as the god of medicine and healing (Woods & Woods, 2008). The powers of Asclepius were so great that he could even bring the dead back to life. Hades, god of the dead, was jealous and complained to Zeus that Asclepius was cheating the kingdom of the dead. Consequently, Asclepius was killed by Zeus with a thunderbolt; however, before he died he gave his healing powers to his two daughters: **Panacea**, goddess of healing, and **Hygeia**, goddess of health (Bates & Winder, 1984). Hygeia was given the power to prevent disease, while Panacea was given the ability to treat disease. The words *hygiene* and *panacea* used today in our language can be traced back to the daughters of the Greek god Asclepius.

Throughout Greece, hundreds of elaborate temples were built to worship the Greek healer, Asclepius. These ancient temples of Asclepius left their symbol as a permanent reminder of the past—known as the **caduceus**. The caduceus is a symbol that shows two snakes braided around a staff. It is representative of the medical profession, and is still commonly used today.

Hippocrates (460–377 B.C.) is credited as the first epidemiologist and the father of modern medicine (Duncan, 1988). Hippocrates developed a theory of disease causation and taught that health was the result of balance, and disease was the result of an imbalance. To the Greeks, the ideal person was completely balanced in mind, body, and spirit. Hippocrates went against conventional thinking that diseases were sent as a punishment from the gods, and looked on the body as having a balance between the four **humors**: blood, phlegm, black bile, and yellow bile (Association for Science Education, 2011). Hippocrates gave his name to the **Hippocratic Oath**, which is still used today by doctors and other health care professionals swearing to practice medicine ethically.

One of Hippocrates's most noteworthy contributions was the distinction between endemic and epidemic diseases. **Epidemiology** is defined as the study of health-event, health-characteristic, or health-determinant patterns in a society (Nutter, 1999). In present epidemiology, **prevalence** is defined as the total number of cases of the risk factor in the population at a given point in time, and **incidence** is a measure of the risk of developing some new condition within a specified period of time (or the number of new cases of the risk factor in the population at a given point in time). An **endemic** is when an infection is maintained in the population without the need for external inputs, such as chickenpox (around in a steady state). An **epidemic** occurs when new cases of a certain disease, in a given population and during a given period of time, substantially exceed what is expected based on recent experience. An epidemic may be restricted to one geographic location; however, if it spreads to other countries or continents and affects a substantial number of people, it is termed a **pandemic,** such as HIV/AIDS (CDC, 2011).

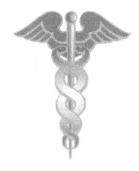

Figure 3.1.   Illustration of a Caduceus.

© Thank You/Shutterstock, Inc.

Romans (500 B.C.–500 A.D.)

The Romans conquered the Mediterranean world, including Greece. The Romans, however, did not destroy many of the health practices and ideas of the Greeks. The Romans placed much emphasis on community health. The Roman Empire built an extensive and efficient aqueduct system, which brought clean water into their cities. Evidence of nearly 200 Roman aqueducts still remains today, from Spain to Syria and from Northern Europe to North Africa (McKenzie, Pinger, & Kotecki, 2008). The Romans also built widespread underground sewers, had extensive bath and wash houses, had a system for getting rid of garbage and other waste, and built the first known hospital. The Romans furthered the work of the Greeks in the study of human anatomy and the practice of surgery. A number of Roman anatomists even dissected living human beings to further their knowledge of the human anatomy (Libby, 1922).

Middle Ages (500–1500)

The era from the collapse of the Roman Empire to 1500 is known as the Middle Ages, or the Dark Ages. The collapse of the Roman Empire resulted in political and social unrest, and many health advances of the time were lost. People went to the opposite extreme and placed little emphasis on cleanliness or hygiene. There was overcrowding and a lack of fresh water; sanitation was ignored and there was waste in the streets; people seldom bathed, and wore perfume to cover up the stench of filthy clothing; diets were poor; it was immoral to view one's own body; and many epidemics took place during this time period (Cottrell et al., 2012).

Christianity was born before the collapse of Rome, but became dominant during the Middle Ages. Both pagan and Christian beliefs blamed disease on supernatural causes. It was a general belief that disease was a judgment from God for sin. This led to a failure to prevent the spread of communicable diseases. The health-related advances of the Greco-Roman era were abandoned and rejected. Entire libraries were burned, and any knowledge concerning the human body was viewed as shameful. This is often referred to as the *Spiritual Era of Public Health.*

The Middles Ages were afflicted by great epidemics. **Leprosy,** one of the earliest recorded epidemic diseases, spread from Egypt to Asia Minor to Europe. Leprosy is a highly contagious and virulent disease characterized by severe facial disfigurement. In some communities, lepers were given the last rites of the church, banished, forced to wear identifying clothing, and required to carry a rod identifying them as lepers. Some lepers were even forced to wear a bell around their neck and ring it as a warning when others came near. Isolated lepers succumbed quickly to starvation and the elements. Inhumane measures ended leprosy in Europe (Goerke & Stebbins, 1968).

Bubonic plague, known as the **Black Death,** may have been the most severe epidemic the world has ever known. The death toll and the disruption of society resulting from the bubonic plague was greater than that from any war, famine, or natural disaster in history. Literally one out of every three or four people contracted the disease and died. Estimates of casualties in Europe vary from 20 to 35 million, with Europe losing one-quarter to one-third of its entire population. Often doctors and religious leaders were some of the first victims, leaving many communities without religious or medical leadership (Cottrell et al., 2012).

Despite the many differences that existed at the time regarding the cause of disease, it was not until the Middle Ages and the epidemics of leprosy and the bubonic plague that the concept of contagion (i.e., disease can be spread from an infected person to a noninfected person) became more universally accepted. This opened the door to interest in science and weakened the sin-disease theory. The Middles Ages also witnessed a number of other communicable diseases, including smallpox, diphtheria, measles, influenza, tuberculosis, anthrax, trachoma, and syphilis (McKenzie et al., 2008).

Renaissance (1500–1700)

The Renaissance, which means "rebirth," was an era characteristic of the Greeks and Romans in which the search for knowledge was revitalized. The experience of the Middle Ages, however, was not forgotten and scientific advances were slow. There was still much disease, and medical care was rudimentary. Bloodletting was a major form of treatment for everything from the common cold to tuberculosis. Animal parts and oils were commonly used as remedies, and examining urine for color changes was a common means of diagnosis. Barbers performed surgery and dentistry because they had the best chairs and sharpest instruments available (Cottrell et al., 2012).

The Renaissance was a period of exploration and expanded trade. Explorers, traders, and colonists took indigenous European diseases and spread them to the indigenous people in the New World. English royalty lived better than the laboring class; however, hygiene and other health-related problems still existed. Disposal of human waste and severe uncleanliness were common problems. Chamber pots were often used and their contents were merely tossed out of the nearest window (ThinkQuest, 2011).

During this era, science emerged again as a legitimate field of inquiry. People now asked how diseases arose and began to think that disease was not a punishment from God. Doctors began to investigate the study of infectious diseases. A Dutch clockmaker, **Antonie Van Leeuwenhoek**, made one of the first microscopes and proved there were life forms too small for the human eye to see. Careful observations led to the recognition of a number of different infections, including cholera, typhoid, tuberculosis, and smallpox. **Andreas Vesalius** and **Leonardo Da Vinci** dissected human bodies and made the first anatomical drawings. As the understanding of the human body increased, so did the development of new medicines. Renaissance apothecaries (pharmacists) experimented with new plants brought from distant lands by explorers, including Christopher Columbus (Association for Science Education, 2011). Figure 3.2 represents the Vitruvian Man, which translates to proportions of the human body, a drawing by Leonardo Da Vinci. The drawing depicts a man in two superimposed positions with his arms and legs apart inscribed in a circle and a square based on the correlations of ideal human proportions with geometry.

Age of Enlightenment (1700s)

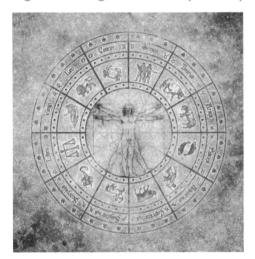

Figure 3.2. Leonardo Da Vinci's Vitruvian Man.

© Shutterstock.com.

The 1700s were a period of revolution, industrialization, and urbanization. Living conditions were poor and overcrowded, water supplies were contaminated, and working conditions were unsafe. Disease and epidemics continued to be a problem. The general belief was that disease was formed in filth and that epidemics were caused by some poisonous vapor or mist filled with particles from decomposed matter (miasmata) that caused illnesses. This concept, known as the **Miasmas Theory**, remained popular until the nineteenth century. A significant milestone for both medicine and public health occurred in 1796, when **Dr. Edward Jenner** demonstrated the process of vaccination as a protection against smallpox. Before this there had been only variolation (inoculation with smallpox material). Jenner's discovery led to an improved understanding of the human immune system and eventual institution of vaccination programs to protect against diseases such as measles, mumps, polio, and tuberculosis (Association for Science Education, 2011).

In the 1700s, health conditions in the United States were similar to those in Europe. A large number of immigrants were entering the ports, cities were growing, and overcrowding existed. Diseases such as smallpox, cholera, and diphtheria were prevalent. Additionally, due to the slave trade, diseases such as yaws, yellow fever, and malaria were common in southern states. The primary means of controlling diseases were quarantines and environmental regulations. In 1789, the first life-expectancy tables (one measure of health status for a given population) were developed by **Dr. Edward Wigglesworth** (Cottrell et al., 2012). The first U.S. census was taken in 1790; life expectancy at birth was only 28 years of age (U.S. National Center for Health Statistics, 2011).

The 1800s

Great advances in the study of biology and bacteria were made during the 1800s. It was realized that social and sanitary conditions impacted the economy. Industrialization led to the concentration of populations in cities. Smallpox, cholera, typhoid, and tuberculosis reached high endemic levels (Pickett & Hanlon, 1990). In 1842, a historical event in public health was witnessed when **Edwin Chadwick** published his *Report on an Inquiry into the Sanitary Conditions of the Laboring Populations of Great Britain* (Cottrell et al., 2012). Chadwick documented the deplorable conditions of the laboring class, and made a strong case that conditions were the cause of disease and suffering. The report called for government intervention and eventually led to the formation of a General Board of Health for England in 1848 (Goerke & Stebbins, 1968).

In the London epidemic of 1854, **Dr. John Snow** mapped out clusters of cholera cases. He identified the source of the cholera outbreak as the public water pump located on Broad Street. His work convinced the local council to disable the well pump by removing its handle, which abated the epidemic in London. In 1862, **Louis Pasteur** proposed the germ theory of disease and introduced the first scientific approach to immunization and then later developed a technique to pasteurize milk. **Robert Koch** became known for isolating *Bacillus anthracis* (1877), the tuberculosis bacillus (1882), and the *Vibrio cholera* (1883), as well as for his development of Koch's postulates. Robert Koch formulated four postulates contributing to germ theory: (1) the disease agent must be found in all cases of the disease, (2) the disease agent must be isolated in a pure culture, (3) inoculation of the disease agent must produce the same disease in healthy animals/people, and (4) the disease agent must be reisolated from the inoculated animal/person (Nobel Lectures, 1967). Between 1877 and the end of the century, many bacteria that caused particular infectious diseases were identified. Consequently, the years from 1875 to 1900 became known as the *Bacteriological Period of Public Health*.

The 1800s in the United States witnessed conditions of overcrowding, poverty, and slow improvement in public health measures. Epidemics were common for smallpox, yellow fever, cholera, typhoid, and typhus; tuberculosis and malaria were endemic (Cottrell et al., 2012). A major report helped to initiate the public health reform movement in the United States, just as Chadwick's landmark 1842 report stimulated public health reform in Britain. In 1805, **Lemuel Shattuck**, a legislator from Massachusetts, published the *Report of the Sanitary Commission of Massachusetts*. The report included remarkable insight about public health issues and the sanitary problems of Massachusetts. This document was ahead of its time, as there still were no national or state public health programs in existence.

Among the many recommendations included in Shattuck's report were: establish state and local boards of health; hire sanitary police or inspectors; collect and analyze vital statistics; implement sanitation programs for towns and buildings; study health of schoolchildren; study, supervise, and/or control TB, alcoholism, and mental disease; supervise and study immigrants; erect model tenements and bath/wash houses; control smoke and food adulteration; establish nursing schools; teach sanitary science in medical school; include prevention in clinical practice; encourage routine physical exams; keep records of family illnesses; and preach health from the pulpit (Odhwani, 2011). The impact of this report jump-started the *Modern Era of Public Health* in America. The Massachusetts State Board of Health was founded in 1869; and by 1900 state health departments existed in 38 states (Cottrell et al., 2012).

The 1900s—America

The time from 1900 to 1960 is known as the *Health Resources Development Period*; and the period from 1900 to 1920 is subcategorized as the *Reform Phase of Public Health*. Many social health problems still existed in the United States, and emphasis was placed on treatment over prevention. In the early 1900s, causes of mortality were mainly from infectious diseases, such as pneumonia and tuberculosis (see Figure 3.3). To address

Rank Order	Cause of death and category numbers of the Fifth Revision of the International Lists		Number	Rate
	1902			
	All causes --		343,217	1,719.1
1	Pneumonia (all forms) and influenza ------------------	107–109, 33	40,362	202.2
2	Tuberculosis (all forms) -------------------------------	13–22	38,820	194.4
3	Diarrhea, enteritis, and ulceration of the intestines --	119, 120	28,491	142.7
4	Diseases of the heart -----------------------------------	90–95	27,427	137.4
5	Intracranial lesions of vascular origin -----------------	83	21,353	106.9
6	Nephritis (all forms) ------------------------------------	130–132	17,699	88.6
7	All accidents --	169–195	14,429	72.3
8	Cancer and other malignant tumors --------------------	45–55	12,769	64.0
9	Senility --	162	10,015	50.2
10	Diphtheria ---	10	8,056	40.3

Source: 1900–1940 tables ranked in National Office of Vital Statistics, December 1947.

Rank[3]	Cause of death (Based on the Tenth Revision, International Classification of Diseases, Second Edition, 2004) and State	Number	Percent of total deaths	Rate
	United States			
...	All causes	2,423,712	100.0	803.6
1	Diseases of heart (I00–I09, I11, I13, I20-I51)	616,067	25.4	204.3
2	Malignant neoplasms (C00–C97)	562,875	23.2	186.6
3	Cerebrovascular diseases (I60–I69)	135,952	5.6	45.1
4	Chronic lower respiratory diseases (J40– J47)	127,924	5.3	42.4
5	Accidents (unintentional injuries) (V01– X59, Y85– Y86)	123,706	5.1	41.0
6	Alzheimer's disease (G30)	74,632	3.1	24.7
7	Diabetes mellitus (E10– E14)	71,382	2.9	23.7
8	Influenza and pneumonia (J09– J18)	52,717	2.2	17.5
9	Nephritis, nephrotic syndrome and nephrosis (N00– N07, N17– N19, N25– N27)	46,448	1.9	15.4
10	Septicemia (A40– A41)	34,828	1.4	11.5
11	Intentional self-harm (suicide) (*U03, X60– X84, Y87.0)	34,598	1.4	11.5
12	Chronic liver disease and cirrhosis (K70, K73– K74)	29,165	1.2	9.7
13	Essential hypertension and hypertensive renal disease (I10,I12,I15)	23,965	1.0	7.9
14	Parkinson's disease (G20– G21)	20,058	0.8	6.7
15	Assault (homicide) (*U01– *U02, X85– Y09, Y87.1)	18,361	0.8	6.1
...	All other causes (Residual)	451,034	18.6	149.5

Source: CDC/NCHS, National Vital Statistics System
[1]Rank based on number of deaths   ...Category not applicable

Figure 3.3. Death Rates in 1900 and 2007.

Table 3.1.   *Healthy People 2020*—Vision, Mission, and Goals.

Vision:

A society in which all people live long, healthy lives.

Mission:

Healthy People 2020 strives to:

• Identify nationwide health improvement priorities.
• Increase public awareness and understanding of the determinants of health, disease, and disability and the opportunities for progress.
• Provide measurable objectives and goals that are applicable at the national, state, and local levels.
• Engage multiple sectors to take actions to strengthen policies and improve practices that are driven by the best available evidence and knowledge.
• Identify critical research, evaluation, and data-collection needs.

Overarching Goals:

• Attain high-quality, longer lives free of preventable disease, disability, injury, and premature death.
• Achieve health equity, eliminate disparities, and improve the health of all groups.
• Create social and physical environments that promote good health for all.
• Promote quality of life, healthy development, and healthy behaviors across all life stages.

Source: Centers for Disease Control and Prevention.

dire public health conditions, the Pure Foods and Drugs Act was passed in 1906. During this period, the first national voluntary health agencies were also formed. The National Association for the Study and Prevention of Tuberculosis was established in 1902, and the American Cancer Society was founded in 1913. From 1930 through World War II, the role of the federal government in social programs expanded. The Social Security Act of 1935 was a significant milestone and the beginning of the federal government's involvement in social issues, including public health. We usually think of social security as a retirement fund or supplement, but the act provided support for state health departments to develop sanitary facilities and improve maternal and child health (Cottrell et al., 2012).

Two major national health agencies were formed during this time. On May 26, 1930, the Ransdell Act converted the Hygienic Laboratory to the National Institute of Health—now called the National Institutes of Health (NIH). The NIH is one of the premier medical research facilities in the world. In 1946, the Communicable Disease Center was established in Atlanta, Georgia, and is now called the Centers for Disease Control and Prevention (CDC). The CDC is one of the leading international epidemiological centers (CDC, 2011).

In 1946, the Hospital Survey and Construction Act, also known as the Hill-Burton Act, was passed to improve the distribution and quality of hospitals (McKenzie et al., 2008). Passage of the Hill-Burton Act led to the rapid construction of new hospitals throughout the nation. Facilities that received funding were required to provide a reasonable volume of free health care to those who could not afford to pay. The Hill-Burton Act placed focus on the medical treatment of disease rather than on public health prevention programs. During this time, there was a shift of emphasis from communicable (**acute**) to noncommunicable (**chronic**) diseases.

The time from 1960 to 1973 is known as the *Period of Social Engineering.* In 1965, the federal government passed legislation designed to improve the health status of the U.S. population. To account for underserved people (the poor and the elderly), Congress passed the Medicare and Medicaid bills as amendments to the Social Security Act of 1935. **Medicare** was constructed to assist in the payment of health care for the elderly; **Medicaid** was designed to provide health insurance for the poor. These bills provided medical care for millions of people who could not otherwise have obtained health care services. Consequently, these bills increased the cost of health care for everyone. This increased access was not necessarily responsible for increasing the costs associated with any given individual's health care. Rather, the problem of health care costs lies within universal price gouging—or charging much more for products and/or services than is reasonable or fair.

Period of Health Promotion (1974—Present)

The *Period of Health Promotion* denotes that the greatest potential for saving lives is in education and lifestyle changes by individuals. Remarkable advancements in public health and health education took place during the latter part of the twentieth century. The U.S. Department of Health and Human Services identified a number of public health achievements which had the greatest impact on the causes of morbidity and mortality during the twentieth century, including an increase in life expectancy, control of major infectious diseases, widespread fluoridation of drinking water, decrease in infant and maternal mortality rates, effective vaccination programs, recognition of tobacco as a health hazard, increase in motor vehicle safety, safer workplaces, and healthier available foods (USDHHS, 1999).

In 1979, the United States government published the first major recognition of the importance of lifestyle in promoting health and well-being, *Healthy People: The Surgeon General's Report on Health Promotion and Disease Prevention* (U.S. Public Health Service, 1979). **Healthy People** is a comprehensive, nationwide health-promotion and disease-prevention agenda designed to serve as a roadmap for improving the health of all people in the United States. In 1980, *Promoting Health/Preventing Disease: Objectives for the Nation* was released. This federal document contained 226 health objectives for the nation, divided into three areas: preventative services, health protection, and health promotion. Although not all health objectives were met, the planning and evaluation process became a valuable way to measure progress of public health in the United States. This led to developing national health objectives for each decade (Cottrell et al., 2012). In 1990, *Healthy People 2000: National Health Promotion and Disease Prevention Objectives* was circulated, and in 2000, *Healthy People 2010: Understanding and Improving Health* was released.

Most recently, in December 2010, *Healthy People 2020* was published. *Healthy People 2020* is committed to a single overarching purpose: promoting health and preventing illness, disability, and premature death (CDC, 2012). *Healthy People 2020* includes a vision statement, a mission statement, four overarching goals (see Table 3.1), and objectives spread over 38 different topic areas (see Table 3.2). *Healthy People* can be used by many different health education and health care professionals, states, communities, professional organizations, and others to help develop intervention programs designed to improve health status.

After a long wait, on October 27, 1997, the Standard Occupational Classification (SOC) Policy Review Committee approved the creation of a new, distinct classification for the occupation of health educator. The recognition of health education and health promotion as a profession is an important historical event in public health. Approval of health education as an occupational classification means the Department of Commerce's Bureau of the Census and other federal agencies now collect data on health education specialists (Cottrell et al., 2012).

As health promotion increased, so did overall life expectancy. In 2007, life expectancy in the United States was the highest in recorded history, reaching 77.9 years of age. By 2020, the projected life expectancy at birth in the United States will be 79.5 years of age (U.S. National Center for Health Statistics, 2011). While public health has made great progress, there is still much to be accomplished. There are many people in the United States and worldwide who do not have access to adequate health care or the information and skills of a professionally trained health education specialist. Public health issues of concern for health educators and other health care professionals in the twenty-first century include lifestyle diseases (heart disease, cancer, stroke, diabetes, and obesity), health care delivery, environmental problems, alcohol and other drug abuse, as well as new communicable diseases or old diseases that have become resistant to drug therapy.

The Profession of Health Education

The Goal of Health Education

As a profession, health education is devoted to employing health promotion processes that foster healthy behaviors. According to the National Commission for Health Education Credentialing (NCHEC, 1996), the goal of health education as a profession is "to promote, maintain, and improve individual and community health. The teaching-learning process is the hallmark and social agenda that differentiates the practice of health education from other helping professions in achieving this goal." The goal of health education is easily identified and explained; however, the role of a health educator can be intricate and challenging. According to the Joint Committee on Health Education and Health Promotion Terminology (2001), a **health educator** is "a professionally prepared individual who serves in a variety of roles and is specifically trained to use appropriate

Table 3.2. *Healthy People 2020—38 Topic Areas.*

Access to Health Services	Heart Disease and Stroke
Adolescent Health	HIV
Arthritis, Osteoporosis, and Chronic Back Conditions	Immunization and Infectious Diseases
	Injury and Violence Prevention
Blood Disorders and Blood Safety	Lesbian, Gay, Bisexual, and Transgender Health
Cancer	Maternal, Infant, and Child Health
Chronic Kidney Disease	Medical Product Safety
Dementias, including Alzheimer's Disease	Mental Health and Mental Disorders
Diabetes	Nutrition and Weight Status
Disability and Health	Occupational Safety and Health
Early and Middle Childhood	Older Adults
Educational and Community-Based Programs	Oral Health
Environmental Health	Physical Activity
Family Planning	Preparedness
Food Safety	Public Health Infrastructure
Genomics	Respiratory Diseases
Global Health	Sexually Transmitted Infections
Health Communication and Health Information Technology	Sleep Health
	Social Determinants of Health
Health-Care-Associated Infections	Substance Abuse
Health-Related Quality of Life & Well-Being	Tobacco Use
Hearing and Other Sensory or Communication Disorders	Vision

Source: Centers for Disease Control and Prevention.

educational strategies and methods to facilitate the development of policies, procedures, interventions, and systems conducive to the health of individuals, groups, and communities." The U.S. Bureau of Labor Statistics (2017) defines health educators as those who "provide and manage health education programs that help individuals, families, and their communities maximize and maintain healthy lifestyles. Collect and analyze data to identify community needs prior to planning, implementing, monitoring, and evaluating programs designed to encourage healthy lifestyles, policies, and environments. May serve as resource to assist individuals, other health professionals, or the community, and may administer fiscal resources for health education programs." Health educators take on a multitude of responsibilities, however, the major role of health educators is to plan, implement, and evaluate health promotion programs.

Target Populations in Health Education

A **target population** is a group of individuals to whom health education programs specifically intend to provide assistance. In the practice of health education, the most common target populations include children, mothers, seniors, minorities, low-income individuals, and disabled individuals. Established in 1975, the WIC (Women, Infants, and Children) program is a health education and promotion program which specifically addresses the needs of women, infants, and children. WIC provides assistance to its target population by providing supplemental foods, health care referrals, and nutrition education (U.S. Department of Agriculture, Food and Nutrition Services, 2011). Additionally, the Institute on Aging provides numerous services for seniors, such as geriatric assessments, home care and support services, community living services, social day programs, psychological counseling, as well as education and training services. (Institute on Aging, 2018).

Following the identification of target populations, health education specialists must identify the risk factors, or the focus, toward which health promotion and disease prevention programming should be aimed. **Risk factors** are defined as "those inherited, environmental, and behavioral influences which are known (or thought) to increase the likelihood of physical or mental problems" (Slee, Slee, & Schmidt, 2008, p. 510). Risk factors are divided into two categories: (1) modifiable (changeable or controllable) and (2) nonmodifiable (unchangeable or uncontrollable). Modifiable risk factors include behaviors such as poor dietary habits, smoking, and sedentary lifestyle. Nonmodifiable risk factors include age, sex, and inherited genes, or factors individuals cannot change or have control over. Both modifiable and nonmodifiable risk factors increase the overall probability of premature morbidity and mortality.

Settings of Health Education

In 1999, Green and Ottoson indicated that the practice of health education was based on the specific assumption "that beneficial health behavior will result from a combination of planned, consistent, integrated learning opportunities. This assumption rests on the scientific evaluations of health education programs in schools, at worksites, in medical settings, and through mass media." While the practice of health education can take place in various environments and institutions, there are four specific settings of health education: schools, communities, worksites, and health care settings. The settings of health education are key because they provide locations for interventions or programs, provide a gateway to target populations, provide necessary communication channels for program distribution, and provide administrative change which can cultivate positive health behaviors (Mullen et al., 1994).

School Health Education

School health education involves educating school-age children and young adults about health and healthy behaviors. According to the American School Health Association (2011), the practice of school health includes "all the strategies, activities, and services offered by, in, or in association with schools that are designed to promote students' physical, emotional, and social development." The goal of health education in schools is to teach students to adopt and maintain lifelong health behaviors, such as hand washing, proper dental care, the importance of exercise, as well as healthy eating habits (Joint Committee on National Health Education Standards, 2007).

In some cases, when school health education is a district-wide concentration, it is known as a coordinated school health program. A **coordinated school health program** is defined as "an organized set of policies, procedures, and activities designed to protect, promote, and improve the health and well-being of students and staff, thus improving a student's ability to learn. It includes, but it is not limited to, comprehensive school health education; school health services; a healthy school environment; school counseling; psychological and social services; physical education; school nutrition services; family and community involvement in school health; and school-site health promotion for staff" (Joint Committee, 2001, p. 99). A coordinated school health program (CSHP) not only focuses on students, but it also benefits school faculty, staff, and administration.

Community Health Education

The Joint Committee on Health Education and Health Promotion Terminology (2001) defines **community health education** as "a theory-driven process that promotes health and prevents disease within populations." The health of a community is the sum total of the health of the individuals who comprise that community. Community health education programs are implemented to target individuals, communities, a state, or the nation. The primary purpose of a community health educator is to plan, implement, or evaluate any health education component within any community outreach program. Typically, community health educators experience more diversity relative to their job duties as compared to the other settings of health education. This is mainly due to the variety of programs created by the various voluntary and public health agencies. Depending upon the need of the agency, community health educators may be responsible for delivering the health promotion program or handling administrative tasks, such as program planning, managing volunteers, and budgeting. Relative to community health education, health educators are typically employed by voluntary health agencies and public health agencies. Voluntary health agencies, such as the American Cancer Society, American Heart Association, and the American Lung Association, address health needs not met by government agencies. Public health agencies, or government health agencies, are supported by tax dollars and include public health departments.

Worksite Health Education

The Joint Committee on Health Education and Health Promotion Terminology (2001) defines **worksite health education** as "a combination of educational, organizational, and environmental activities designed to improve the health and safety of employees and their families." Worksite health education and promotion programs vary greatly depending upon the organization. Some companies may offer discounts to fitness facilities, while other organizations own fitness facilities specifically designed for employee use. The duties of a worksite health educator can range from providing tutorials on smoking cessation, stress management, workplace safety, and cancer risk awareness to assessing employees' overall health status by checking their blood pressure and cholesterol levels. If the worksite health promotion program is based within the company's fitness center, employers may desire worksite health educators to have training in exercise testing or exercise prescription (Cottrell et al., 2009). Additionally, training in first aid and CPR is another desirable skill for worksite health educators, especially if they work in a fitness center.

Worksite health promotion programs focused on prevention and interventions that reduce employees' health risk factors are beneficial for both the employee and the employer. While unhealthy behavior and lifestyle greatly affect an individual's health, it can also directly impact the employer's compensation and health care costs. Healthy employees save organizations money, as they are less likely to call in sick, less likely to utilize health care services, have fewer work-related injuries, and are, overall, more productive. Moreover, these health intervention programs can positively boost employee morale, which in turn results in less employee turnover. Figure 3.4 illustrates selected means and methods of protection in the workplace.

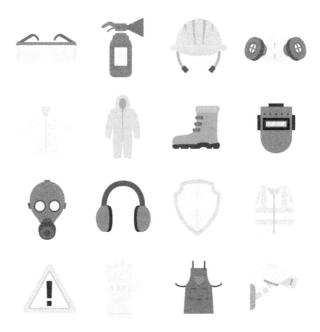

Figure 3.4.   Worksite Safety.

© Shutterstock.com.

Health Care Health Education

Health care settings include public (not-for-profit) hospitals, for-profit hospitals, medical care clinics, home health agencies, health maintenance organizations (HMOs), and preferred provider organizations (PPOs) (Breckon, Harvey, & Lancaster, 1998). "Typically in the medical care field, health educators serve as administrators, directors, managers, and coordinators, supporting and consulting on health education programs and services" (Totzkay-Sitar & Cornett, 2007). This is mostly because health insurance companies do not provide reimbursement for the services of a health educator; therefore, the duty of patient education falls heavily upon the nursing staff who are not trained in the same manner as a health education specialist (Cottrell, Girvan, & McKenzie, 2009). Additionally, it is common for health educators to oversee fitness programs for hospital employees or patients (Breckon et al., 1998). These fitness programs may specifically be designed for "in house" use only, or could be open to the community as an outreach program. Essentially, health education and promotion programs in health care settings are similar to those in worksite health education and promotion. What differentiates them is that health care settings generally encompass outreach programs and patient education programs.

Summary

Since ancient times, humans have been searching for techniques to be healthy and disease free. Early humans relied heavily on superstition and spiritualism as remedies for disease. The early civilizations of Egypt, Greece, and Rome experienced great progress in public health. This is evident through systems of waste disposal, safer drinking water, and the inception of pharmacology. However, during the Middle Ages, society took a step backward and much of the knowledge gained was lost. Science was rejected, while religion gained favor as the means of preventing and treating disease. The Renaissance was a period of rebirth, in which interest in science and knowledge reemerged. The Age of Enlightenment witnessed growth in cities, and the Industrial Revolution took place in both England and the United States. Sanitation problems, overcrowding, and epidemics were still prevalent. Public health in the United States emerged in the mid-1850s and 1900s. Health departments were established at local, city, and state levels. Professional organizations and voluntary health agencies were formed. During the 1960s, two major pieces of government legislation (Medicare and Medicaid) were passed to improve health conditions among the elderly and the poor. By the 1970s, health care costs had escalated, and concern had shifted from treatment to prevention. This led to the development of national health objectives for the decades of the 1980s, 1990s, 2000, 2010, and 2020. Health education and health promotion emerged as an official profession. Overall life expectancy has increased as health promotion has improved; however, there is still much progress to be accomplished in the future of public health.

Health is a dynamic process that is always changing based upon an individual's lifestyle and environment. The eight dimensions of wellness address each aspect of life which has an impact on an individual's overall well-being. If one dimension of wellness is not fulfilled the wheel will be off-balance, and therefore, it cannot function to its true potential. Health behavior includes three categories: preventative health behavior, illness behavior, and sick-role behavior. Health promotion consists of three main pillars: good governance, health literacy, and healthy cities. Health education emphasizes three levels of prevention: primary prevention, secondary prevention, and tertiary prevention. Health educators are responsible for helping individuals facilitate health-conscious behaviors by planning, implementing, and evaluating health promotion programs. Health education may take place in various environments, however, the practice of health education is most common in schools, communities, worksites, and health care settings. As the profession of health education continues to expand, thoughts of the future must be in the forefront. It is necessary for government policy makers to continually reevaluate and create new environmental and social standards which are most conducive to the health and well-being of society.

References

Association for Science Education. (2011). *History of medicine.* Retrieved from http://resources.schoolscience. co.uk/abpi/history/history4.html.

Bates, I. J., & Winder, A. E. (1984). *Introduction to health education.* San Francisco: Mayfield.

Centers for Disease Control and Prevention (CDC). (2011). *Principles of Epidemiology* (2nd ed.). Atlanta. Retrieved from http://www2a.cdc.gov/phtn/catalog/pdf-file/Epi_course.pdf.

Centers for Disease Control and Prevention (CDC). (2012). *Healthy People 2020.* Retrieved from http://www. cdc.gov/nchs/healthy_people/hp2020.htm.

Cottrell, R., Girvan, J., & McKenzie, J. (2012). *Principles and foundations of health promotion and education.* San Francisco: Pearson Education/Benjamin Cummings.

Duncan, D. (1988). *Epidemiology: Basis for disease prevention and health promotion.* New York: Macmillan.

Green, W. H., & Simons-Morton, B. G. (1990). *Introduction to health education.* Prospect Heights, IL: Waveland Press.

Goerke, L. S., & Stebbins, E. L. (1968). *Mustard's introduction to health education.* Prospect Heights, IL: Macmillan.

Health Guidance. (2011). *Ancient Hebrew Medicine.* Retrieved from http://www.healthguidance.org/entry/ 6309/1/Ancient-Hebrew-Medicine.html.

Libby, W. (1922). *The history of medicine in its salient features.* Boston: Houghton Mifflin.

McKenzie, J. F., Pinger, R. R., & Kotecki, J. E. (2008). *An introduction to community health* (6th ed.). Boston: Jones & Bartlett.

Nobel Lectures. (1967). *Physiology or Medicine, 1901–1921.* Amsterdam: Elsevier.

Nutter, F. W. (1999). Understanding the interrelationships between botanical, human, and veterinary epidemiology: the Ys and Rs of it all. *Ecosystem Health,* 5, 131–140.

Odhwani, A. (2011). *Public Health: Historical Perspective.* PowerPoint Lecture.

Pickett, G., & Hanlon, J. (1990). *Public health administration and practice* (9th ed.). St. Louis: Times Mirror.

ThinkQuest. (2011). *Renaissance Medicine.* Retrieved from http://library.thinkquest.org/15569/hist-7.html.

U.S. Department of Health and Human Services (USDHHS). (1999). Changes in the public health system. *Morbidity and Mortality Weekly Report, 50,* 1141.

U.S. National Center for Health Statistics. (2011). QuickStats: Life expectancy at birth, by race and sex—United States, 2000–2009. *Morbidity and Mortality Weekly Report, 60,* 588.

U.S. Public Health Service. (1979). *Healthy people: The surgeon general's report on health promotion and disease prevention.* Washington, DC: U.S. Government Printing Office.

Woods, M., & Woods, M. (2008). *Seven wonders of ancient Greece.* Minneapolis: Twenty-first Century Books.

Chapter 3—Review Questions

1. Compare and contrast the health practices of the early Egyptians with modern-day health care and health education practices.

2. Identify three major contributions the Greeks provided to health care and public health.

3. What were the major epidemics of the Middle Ages? How did these epidemics contribute to a change in beliefs regarding the spread of disease?

4. Discuss the important contributions to health care that occurred during the Renaissance.

5. How did Dr. Edward Jenner's research play a part in the modern-day immunization process?

6. Identify four individuals who made major contributions to health and health care in the 1800s. What are these individuals known for?

7. What did the Social Security Act of 1935 mean for Americans? Also, what was the purpose of the Medicare and Medicaid bills which amended the Social Security Act of 1935?

8. Compare and contrast the leading causes of death in 1900 and 2005 relative to contraction or development.

9. Explain the evolution of *Healthy People* and why it is important to health education.

10. Identify the major health concerns for the twenty-first century and discuss some health education measures which could be taken to combat these concerns.

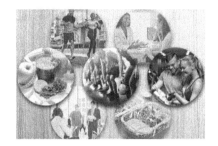

CHAPTER 4
Introduction to Theory and the Health Belief Model

art II of this book focuses specifically on intrapersonal theories: Health Belief Model (HBM); Theory of Reasoned Action (TRA)/Theory of Planned Behavior (TPB); and the Transtheoretical Model (TTM) and Stages of Change. Theory provides a basic foundation from which health educators can build evidence-based interventions. However, in order to use theory effectively, it is imperative to understand the underlying terms related to theoretical frameworks. The present chapter provides definitions for the basic terminology as applied to health education/promotion theory, covers content on the social ecological perspective, and explores the Health Belief Model (HBM), one of the most widely used models for understanding health behavior.

Introduction

As an introduction to intrapersonal theories, consider your own personal health behaviors for a moment. Why do you or do you not exercise, eat nutritiously, wear a seat belt, follow your doctor's recommendations, and drink diet or regular soda? To what extent do your behaviors depend on your attitudes? Which attitudes are most important? Now consider the possibility of initiating a new behavior, or a behavior different from what you have been doing, such as a new exercise routine or a new diet. What factors would influence the likelihood of your adopting this new behavior? Which factors are most influential?

Attitude-oriented theories, also known as expectancy value theories, are influential in health promotion because attitudes are not fixed. They evolve over time with new experiences and the introduction of new information. By identifying the attitudes and beliefs associated with health behavior, it is possible to provide new information that can alter these dispositions with predictable effect on behavior. Of course, information comes from many sources, including everyday-life events and experiences as well as incidental and purposeful messages. **Expectancy value theories** were developed to explain how individuals' behaviors are influenced by beliefs and attitudes toward objects and actions (Simons-Morton, McLeroy, & Wendel, 2012). They provide comprehensive explanations of the beliefs and attitudes that underlie behavior. This group of theories assumes people behave according to the personal benefits an action is anticipated or expected to provide, considering the benefits and costs of the alternatives. Expectancy value theories suggest that behavior is most likely to occur when the advantages (benefits) of a particular action outweigh the costs (barriers).

Definitions

Prior to learning about specific theories used in health education, it is important to first understand the relevant terminology. Following are the definitions for some key terms which describe the important elements in the theories discussed in this chapter and throughout the book. The concepts of knowledge and belief are related, but are not the same. **Knowledge** is information that is factual and verifiable (an objectively verifiable truth). It is what is true—what one can be relatively sure about, anyhow. People, however, sometimes think they know something to be true, but it turns out not to be true. **Beliefs** are what we think is true based on the information we have at hand and our interpretation of it. Beliefs are based not only on information, but also on perceptions.

Perceptions are how a person views or interprets information from various sources. For example, two people may obtain the same information or witness the same event, but perceive or interpret it in a completely different fashion.

Attitudes are mindsets established upon an individual's evaluation of an object, thing, or situation. "Attitudes convey an emotional quality that beliefs do not necessarily convey" (Simons-Morton et al., 2012, p. 102). The strength of various attitudes toward a health behavior is significant. The value of an attitude is measured by its strength or importance. This is the reason for response options on attitude questionnaires, such as "strongly agree, agree, disagree, or strongly disagree (SA-SD)." **Values** are defined as the evaluation of the relative importance of various factors, concepts, and actions. Values are more general and are made up of related attitudes. People hold values for small and personal concepts, such as food preferences, chosen occupation, exercise habits, social and leisure activity choices, how one spends their time and money, as well as bigger concepts such as religion and politics. It is possible to simultaneously value free time and work, exercise and watching television, smoking and health; however, many of our decisions are based on measuring or valuing the alternatives. Expectancy value theory is so named because it assumes people tend to behave in ways that they expect will maximize the likelihood of achieving something they value.

A **theory** is defined as "a set of interrelated concepts, definitions, and propositions that present a systematic view of events or situations by specifying relations among variables, in order to explain and predict the events or situations" (Glanz, Rimer, & Viswanath, 2008). Simply stated, a theory provides a general explanation as to why people do and do not behave in certain ways. More specifically related to health education, a theory can explain why an individual chooses to participate or not participate in health-protective behaviors. Theory is often utilized within the profession of health education during various stages of planning, implementing, and evaluating health promotion programs.

Theories are "tools to help health educators better understand what influences health-relevant individuals, groups, and institutional behaviors–and to thereupon plan effective interventions directed at health-beneficial results" (Hochbaum, Sorenson, & Lorig, 1992). "Behavioral and social science theory provides a platform for understanding why people engage in health-risk or health-compromising behavior and why they adopt health-protective behavior" (Crosby, Kegler, & DiClemente, 2002). "A theory based approach provides direction and justification for program activities and serves as a basis for processes that are to be incorporated into the health promotion program" (Cowdery, Wang, Eddy, & Trucks, 1995).

Theories can assist health educators in creating goals and objectives which are appropriate for different types of interventions. Use of theory can also ensure congruency between the planned intervention and expected outcomes of the intervention (McKenzie, Neiger, & Smeltzer, 2005). "Theory is not a substitute for professional judgment, but it can assist health educators in professional decision making. Insofar as the application of theory to practice strengthens program justification, promotes the effective and efficient use of resources, and improves accountability, it also assists in establishing professional credibility" (D'Onofrio, 1992). For example, behavior-change interventions are challenging to create and implement. A health educator may waste valuable time and resources trying to get the participants to achieve behavior change. Therefore, health educators should base their intervention programs upon theories which have proven to be successful in previous interventions with specific target populations who are receptive and who would benefit from the health program.

The primary building blocks of a theory are known as concepts. **Concepts** are the major components of theory; however, when concepts are created or adopted for specific use in a theory, they are called constructs. Therefore, **constructs** are the key concepts which compose theories. When a theory is used in practice, variables are utilized to measure the constructs of the theory for that specific application. **Variables** are the "empirical counterparts or operational forms of constructs" (Glanz et al., 2008). It is very important for variables to be matched with constructs when evaluating theory-based interventions. For example, a health educator who is conducting a smoking-cessation program may be interested in determining whether the Health Belief Model (HBM) could predict which participants will continue to abstain from tobacco use three months after completing the cessation program. To do this, a health educator would focus on the HBM construct of self-efficacy. In order to measure the participants' self-efficacy relative to abstaining from tobacco use, the health educator could utilize a questionnaire including items which address long-term tobacco cessation.

Models are considered a subclass of a theory. **Models** "are generalized, hypothetical descriptions, often based on an analogy, used to analyze or explain something" (Glanz & Rimer, 1995). Models are typically formed from multiple theories and empirical research findings (Earp & Ennett, 1991). A model does not attempt to explain the processes underlying learning, but only represent them.

Social Ecological Perspective

Early attention to health behavior and its role in chronic disease prevention focused on personal choice and life-style behaviors, which were largely believed to be under the control of the individual. In the 1980s, however, literature began to emerge which challenged the personal-choice perspective and began to place individual behavior within a broader social context. Behavior was redefined as representing not only a person's individual choices, but also the person's previous experiences which influenced the choices, the others with whom the person has or had significant relationships, social norms and values, and the social environment in which the person interacts, such as school, work, neighborhoods, communities, and the broader culture (Simons-Morton et al., 2012).

As described by Bronfenbrenner (1979) in *The Ecology of Human Development*, individual behavior may be viewed as occurring within multiple systems. These systems range from the microsystem of the individual and the individual's knowledge, attitudes, values, and life experiences, as well as families and social relationships, to broader meso- (organizational), exo- (community), and macro- (culture) systems. Multiple levels of influence exist at each societal level. For example, each social system affects what people believe and how people behave and, equally important, the effects people have on those systems. Each level is linked to a body of knowledge, discipline, or area of practice. For health educators, this information can provide specific theoretical and empirical analysis of how each level can influence personal health behavior. The **social ecological perspective** comprises a seven-level framework, including (1) intrapersonal, (2) interpersonal, (3) organizational, (4) community, (5) public policy, (6) physical environment, and (7) culture. Figure 4.1 illustrates the relationships of the societal levels in the social ecological perspective.

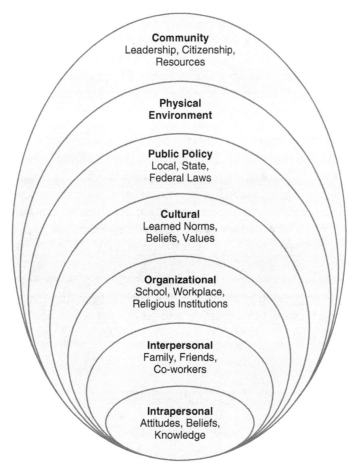

Figure 4.1.   Social Ecological Perspective.

Intrapersonal Level

Individual factors or theories help us understand how individual characteristics (intrapersonal level) may affect behaviors. **Intrapersonal** models and theories are concerned with factors within an individual, such as attitudes, beliefs, experiences, knowledge, motivation and behaviors (Rimer & Glanz, 2005). Intrapersonal theories are mainly concerned with cognitions, dispositions, and contingencies that affect individual behavior. Without question, a person's knowledge, skills, beliefs, perceptions, attitudes, and values are all related to health behavior. For example, individuals who have positive attitudes toward tobacco use are more likely to smoke cigarettes.

Intrapersonal models are divided into two categories: continuum theories and stage theories. **Continuum theories**, such as the Health Belief Model (HBM) and the Theory of Reasoned Action (TRA)/Theory of Planned Behavior (TPB), identify factors which influence behavior and calculate the probability that an individual will take a given action (Weinstein, Rothman, & Sutton, 1998). Continuum theories place individuals along a continuum based upon their likelihood of action. Depending on which of the different variables is most influential, an individual may move either way along the continuum as the likelihood of action changes. **Stage theories**, such as the Transtheoretical Model (TTM), categorize individuals into ordered stages and identify factors which could induce movement from stage to stage (Weinstein & Sandman, 2002a). Stage theories contain four basic principles: (1) a category system to define the stages, (2) an ordering of stages, (3) people in the same stage face common barriers to behavioral change, and (4) people in different stages face different barriers to behavioral change (Weinstein & Sandman, 2002b).

Interpersonal Level

An individual's knowledge, attitudes, values, and beliefs are also influenced by his or her relationships with others and others' attitudes and behaviors. The **interpersonal** level of the social ecological model focuses primarily on interpersonal influences on behavior, such as family, friends, acquaintances, neighbors, and co-workers, as well as the social norms that exist within specific social groups (Simons-Morton et al., 2012). A variety of theories and models have been used to understand interpersonal influences, including those that deal with social roles, social networks, social support, and social influences. For example, adolescent tobacco use is influenced by the information adolescents receive from other people (interpersonal influences), including whether others think they should smoke and the individual's receptiveness to the influence of others.

Organizational Level

Most people spend a significant amount of time within specific community organizations or settings. These organizations include school, workplace, religious institutions, recreational or entertainment facilities, and health care settings. Due to the amount of time we spend in organizations, organizational-level influences exist and play an important role in health promotion and disease prevention activities. Organizations that are of particular importance to health promotion include worksites, schools, churches, health care providers, recreational settings, and community-based organizations (Poland, Green, & Rootman, 2000). These organizational settings provide the opportunity to reach large groups of people and bring forth multiple resources to bear in efforts to improve the health of organizational members (Simons-Morton et al., 2012). Organizations may provide direct services to their members, such as smoking-cessation and weight-loss programs, or they may provide insurance or other coverage for health promotion services. Organizations also set standards for their members and participate in broader community-wide efforts to provide health promotion services to improve the health of the community.

Community Level

A variety of community-level characteristics, including social and community factors, are important in community-based health promotion interventions. These include leadership, citizen participation, resources, skills, interpersonal networks, as well as community history, power, values, and the ability to reflect on community problems and solutions. Major objectives of community-based interventions include community change and building capacity to address community health problems (McLeroy, Norton, Kegler, Burdine, & Sumaya, 2003). For example, there has been a dramatic increase in health promotion programs, including smoking cessation, physical activity, and safety programs carried out by community organizations, such as churches, health care clinics, YMCAs, and other local or state cancer and heart disease associations. The community level of the ecological perspective also works to target social conditions, such as unemployment, poverty, housing, gangs/violence, drug and alcohol use, physical inactivity, obesity, school drop out, as well as adolescent pregnancy and STIs.

Public Policy

Public policy refers to local, state, and federal laws, as well as their regulation, interpretation, and enforcement, that support healthy actions and practices for disease prevention, early detection, control, and management (Simons-Morton et al., 2012). In the case of public health, such laws and interpretations can range from laws requiring seat belt use to tax policies, such as those governing the price and availability of tobacco. In recent years, there has been increasing attention and effort to influence the development, adoption, and application of policy to accomplish health goals. For example, relative to tobacco use, substantial effort has been exercised to influence the implementation of policies to ban smoking in public places, raise the tax on tobacco products, ban the sale of tobacco products to minors, increase the price of health and life insurance for those who use tobacco products, restrict tobacco advertising, and add warning labels on tobacco products. While there is variation in the effectiveness of specific policies, tobacco use among the U.S. population has been reduced by more than 50% since the 1960s (Fiore & Baker, 2009). Policy approaches are now the object of health promotion efforts to address obesity, lack of physical activity, motor vehicle safety, unintentional injuries, and other major public health issues.

Physical Environment

A healthy physical environment is an important goal that can be addressed at many societal levels. There are multiple ways through which the physical (and social) environment may affect health and behavior. According to Stokols (1996), the physical environment may (1) serve as a medium for transmitting infections and diseases, including both air and waterborne diseases; (2) serve as a source of stress through noise, population density, or physical threats; (3) serve as a source of safety or danger through environmental contamination or unsafe areas; (4) serve as an enabler of health behaviors, such as proximity to physical fitness facilities; and (5) provide health resources, such as sanitation systems. The physical environment may affect health directly, through exposure to toxic chemicals, infectious diseases, dangerous settings, or more indirectly through people's perceptions of the physical environment as threatening, safe, or unsafe (Simons-Morton et al., 2012). According to the Transportation Research Board (2005), our physical environment is linked to many risk factors for chronic diseases, such as obesity and diabetes. Characteristics of the physical environment that have been associated with physical activity include land use (population, employment, diversity), accessibility (distance from destinations), design (neighborhood aesthetics), and transportation infrastructure (presence of sidewalks, mass transit, street design).

Cultural Level

The cultural level of the social ecological model is widely used in many disciplines, including public health, health promotion, community psychology, organizational development, health communication, marketing, and program evaluation. Culture has been defined as "a shared system of learned norms, beliefs, values and behaviors that differ across populations defined by region, nationality, ethnicity, or religions" (Hruschka & Hadley, 2008, p. 947). Culture can affect health and health behavior in a variety of ways, including how people think and talk about health problems. Culture affects habits and practices that increase or decrease risk factors for disease, such as hand washing. Culture can also influence health through shared beliefs, attitudes, norms, and values. For example, in the last 50 years, our culture has witnessed a dramatic paradigm shift in the way we view tobacco use. Tobacco is no longer viewed or marketed as a positive, sexually appealing adult behavior; rather it is viewed as a negative behavior practiced by individuals who lack the willpower to quit. Culture is also important in health promotion as the United States has become more multicultural. It has been shown that different cultures have more risk factors or fewer risk factors for certain diseases based on unique patterns of beliefs, practices, attitudes, and values. In the practice of public health and health promotion, it is imperative that health education specialists develop programs and codes of conduct that are appropriate for the target populations being served as well as the cultural system within which the intervention is being conducted.

History of the Health Belief Model

In the 1950s, social psychologists strived to understand behavior by using an approach which incorporated two learning theories: Stimulus Response Theory (Watson, 1925) and Cognitive Theory (Tolman, 1932). **Stimulus Response Theory** indicates that "learning results from events that reduce physiological drives that activate behavior" (Champion & Skinner, 2008). In 1938, Skinner hypothesized that frequency of behavior is directly related to the consequences or reinforcements of the behavior, which is known as operant conditioning (Skinner, 1938). Skinner believed that reasoning and thinking were not required to explain behavior, but rather a system of rewards and punishments provided sufficient means to predict behavior.

Cognitive Theory emphasizes "the role of subjective hypotheses and expectations held by individuals, believing that behavior is a function of the subjective *value* of an outcome and of the subjective probability, or *expectation*, that a particular action will achieve that outcome" (Champion & Skinner, 2008). Cognitive Theory includes reasoning, thinking, and information processing as important components of behavior, whereby they influence the expectations of a situation, not behavior directly. By evolving both the Stimulus Response Theory and the Cognitive Theory to fit the context of health-related behaviors, the two basic assumptions of the Health Belief Model were established: (1) people do not want to become ill, and (2) people expect specific health behaviors to prevent illness.

The **Health Belief Model** (HBM) was created in the 1950s to explain why people were not taking advantage of disease screening programs (Rosenstock, 1960). The HBM was used, initially, to study the perceptions of individuals regarding their susceptibility to tuberculosis and any perceived benefits they would derive from early-detection screenings (Hochbaum, 1958). The model was expanded to incorporate the study of people's reactions to symptoms of disease or illness (Kirscht, 1974) and their behavior after they received a disease diagnosis (Becker, 1974). Since its creation, the HBM continues to be the most widely utilized model to explain health behaviors (Janz & Becker, 1984). Figure 4.2 provides an illustration of the constructs which comprise the HBM.

Constructs of the HBM

The HBM constructs are useful within multiple professions concerned with behavior change. The constructs of the HBM incorporate individual perceptions, which are strong indicators as to whether an individual will prevent, screen for, or control illness (Champion & Skinner, 2008). The HBM is comprised of six constructs: (1) perceived susceptibility, (2) perceived severity, (3) perceived benefits, (4) perceived barriers, (5) cues to action, and (6) self-efficacy.

Perceived Susceptibility

Perceived susceptibility is one's perception of the likelihood that one will contract a disease or illness. Individual perceptions vary across a large continuum. Those at one end deny the possibility of contracting an illness; those at the opposite end admit the possibility of contracting an illness. For example, an individual who perceives the chance of contracting a STI during sexual activity as high is more likely to use a condom compared to someone who perceives contracting a STI as low.

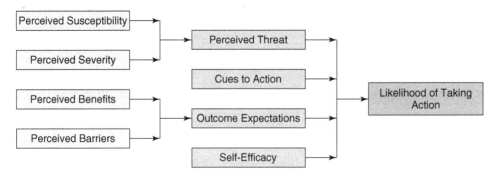

Figure 4.2.   Health Belief Model.

Perceived Severity

Perceived severity refers to the perception of the seriousness of contracting an illness, especially if left untreated. Factors such as pain, discomfort, disability, work restrictions, and interference with social activities account for the perceived seriousness of an illness. Perceived severity is often used in fear marketing strategies to change behavior, such as commercials about local rates of sexually transmitted infections (STIs) and/or unwanted pregnancies. Both perceived severity and perceived susceptibility contribute to the concept of perceived threat. **Perceived threat**, while it is not specifically a construct of the HBM, is a measure which contributes to an individual's likelihood of participating in health-protective behaviors (CHIRr, 2018).

Perceived Benefits

Perceived benefits are the benefits an individual perceives as deriving from participation in health-protective behaviors. For example, benefits we could experience from eating healthfully include feeling better about ourselves and fitting more comfortably into our clothes. At the opposite end, an individual who does not believe a health-protective behavior will reduce susceptibility to disease or illness is less likely to participate in the behavior.

Perceived Barriers

Perceived barriers are any perceived negative consequences which persuade an individual not to participate in a health-protective behavior. Barriers to health-protective behaviors include pain, monetary costs, time, embarrassment, and inconvenience. For example, an individual may choose not to quit smoking because the cost of nicotine patches is too expensive. Typically, individuals consider the perceived benefits minus the perceived barriers when determining their health behavior choice. If the benefits outweigh the barriers, an individual is likely to participate in a health-protective behavior. However, if the barriers outweigh the benefits, the individual is highly unlikely to adopt the health behavior. This mental calculation of benefits minus barriers is known as **outcome expectations**. Outcome expectations is not a construct of the HBM, but when considered with perceived threat, researchers can predict likelihood of action. Table 4.1 provides an example of how outcome expectations are derived.

Cues to Action

Cues to action are triggers which cause an individual to take action and participate in health-protective behaviors. Cues to action include billboards, media stories, friends, family, and internal motivators. It is difficult to study cues to action because of the near-impossibility of pinpointing the exact trigger to action. For example, after long contemplation, you decide to get a flu shot. Did you get the flu shot because (1) your grandmother got one, (2) your roommate just contracted the flu, (3) you saw a warning on the news about the spread of the

Table 4.1.   Example of Outcome Expectations

Calculation of Outcome Expectations for Exercising		
Perceived Benefits of Exercise − Perceived Barriers to Exercise = Taking Action		
Looking "good"	Cost of membership	Begins Exercising
Having more energy	Takes time	
Better sleep		
Self-confidence		
Perceived Benefits of Exercise − Perceived Barriers to Exercise = Not Taking Action		
Looking "good"	Cost of membership	Does Not Begin Exercising
Self-confidence	Takes time	
	No instant results	
	Injuries	

flu in your area, or (4) the flu shot was free? Any one of the four scenarios, or possibly all of them combined, could have contributed to your decision to get a flu shot.

Self-Efficacy

Initially, self-efficacy was not a construct of the HBM. Rosenstock, Strecher, and Becker (1988) suggested that self-efficacy should be added to the HBM as a separate construct. Bandura (1997) defined **self-efficacy** as "the conviction that one can successfully execute the behavior required to produce the outcomes." In other words, it is your confidence in your own ability to participate in a behavior change. While there are measures of generalized self-efficacy, for the purposes of the HBM, think of self-efficacy as task specific. Thus, an individual may possess higher self-efficacy for playing golf as compared to playing basketball.

Other Variables

Other variables, such as age, gender, education, socioeconomic status, and social demographics, can influence an individual's perceptions. While it is almost impossible to control for all of these variables in research, it is still important to realize there are other variables besides the HBM constructs which influence perceptions and behaviors.

HBM as Applied to Tobacco Use

The following is an example of how the HBM may be applied within the "real world." While opening a newly purchased pack of cigarettes, an individual stops to look at the surgeon general's warning on the side of the pack. The warning on the side of the cigarette pack is considered a *cue to action* because it is meant to make the individual contemplate whether to continue to smoke cigarettes. Later, when this individual is at home watching television, a TRUTH campaign commercial broadcasts a message about the negative health consequences related to cigarette smoking. After seeing the TRUTH commercial, another *cue to action*, the individual determines their *perceived susceptibility* of developing lung cancer. After the individual considers how long they have been smoking cigarettes and their daily cigarette consumption, the individual determines they are at high risk for developing lung cancer. Additionally, this individual believes lung cancer is a serious disease, which establishes *perceived severity*. Based upon the individual's perceived susceptibility and perceived severity of lung cancer, the individual is concerned about developing lung cancer (perceived threat).

This individual knows that after 10 years of being cigarette free, the lungs heal and the probability of developing lung cancer reduces greatly (*perceived benefit*). The individual is enthusiastic about quitting smoking and believes they will quit this time (*self-efficacy*). However, in order to quit smoking cigarettes, the individual requires nicotine replacement therapy. At this point in time, the individual is unable to afford the extra expense of the nicotine patches (*perceived barrier*). This individual needs to analyze the perceived benefits of quitting smoking with the perceived barriers of quitting smoking to determine the likelihood of taking action and actually quitting cigarette smoking. Table 4.2 illustrates the constructs of the HBM as applied to cigarette smoking.

Table 4.2. Health Belief Model - Constructs and Examples Applied to Tobacco Use

Cues to Action	Surgeon General's warning TRUTH commercial
Perceived Susceptibility	Length of time as a smoker Amount of daily cigarette consumption
Perceived Severity	Seriousness of lung cancer
Perceived Benefits	After 10 years of being tobacco free Probability of lung cancer greatly decreases
Perceived Barriers	Unable to afford nicotine patches
Self-Efficacy	Confidence in being able to quit smoking
Likelihood of Action	(Perceived Benefits − Perceived Barriers)

Table 4.3. Health Belief Model Constructs and Example Questionnaire Items

Perceived Susceptibility	Tobacco use causes over 400,000 people in the U.S. to die each year. (SA-SD)
Perceived Severity	Smoking-facilitated diseases, such as lung cancer and heart disease, are costly to treat and can cause death. (SA-SD)
Perceived Benefits	The benefits of not smoking cigarettes clearly outweigh any benefits that might be attributed to smoking. (SA-SD)
Perceived Barriers	Factors such as stress, anxiety, and the cost of nicotine patches prevent me from quitting tobacco use. (SA-SD)
Cues to Action	Most people my age smoke cigarettes. (SA-SD)
Self-Efficacy	I believe I can say no to smoking, even if my friends pressure me to smoke. (SA-SD)

Between 1974 and 1984, a review of the HBM was conducted in order to assess its overall performance as a model (Becker, 1974; Janz & Becker, 1984). The review provided a substantial amount of empirical support for the HBM and its performance in predicting behavior. The perceived-barriers construct was found to be the strongest predictor of behavior in all of the studies reviewed. The perceived-severity construct was the least powerful predictor of preventive health behavior; however, perceived severity was strongly correlated with sick-role behavior. Perceived susceptibility was a stronger predictor for preventive behavior than sick-role behavior; whereas, perceived benefits was a stronger predictor for sick-role behavior than preventative behavior. The HBM model is limited because it lacks an emotional component of behavior—fear. Witte believed fear was a strong emotional predictor of behavior because it is a negative emotion which leads to a highly aroused state (Witte, 1992). Fear-based health communications have been identified as a means to affect perceived susceptibility and perceived severity of disease (Baranowski, Cullen, Nicklas, Thompson, & Baranowski, 2003). Adding an emotional construct to the HBM could help explain the correlations between all of the HBM constructs (Rogers & Prentice-Dunn, 1997).

Additionally, the constructs of the HBM can provide limitations within their application due to variability in how the constructs are measured. When applying the HBM to an intervention, it is important to maintain the original definitions of the constructs, utilize behavior-specific measures, and ensure the behaviors are relevant to the target population. Additionally, researchers should create scales or questionnaires which contain multiple measures (at least three items) for each construct in order to include all relevant components of the constructs and reduce measurement error. Table 4.3 provides example questionnaire items which could be utilized to measure the HBM constructs for a tobacco intervention.

Summary

This chapter provided definitions for the basic terminology as applied to health promotion theory and application. Health education specialists should strive to use theory as the foundation for their health promotion programs. Not only does theory provide a starting point during the program-planning stage, but it also provides credibility for any intervention program. It is important for health educators to choose an appropriate theory based upon the type of intervention they create so as to establish a solid theoretical framework which matches the intervention. Content on the social ecological perspective was provided in this chapter and included the levels of (1) intrapersonal, (2) interpersonal, (3) organizational, (4) community, (5) public policy, (6) physical environment, and (7) culture. The second half of the chapter highlighted the Health Belief Model (HBM), one of the most widely utilized intrapersonal models. The HBM is an expectancy value theory. The HBM was created based upon two popular learning theories (Stimulus Response Theory and Cognitive Theory) and has evolved into a model concerned with predictors of health behavior. The HBM is composed of six constructs: perceived susceptibility, perceived severity, perceived benefits, perceived barriers, cues to action, and self-efficacy. All constructs should be taken into consideration when applying the HBM to a health promotion intervention.

References

Bandura, A. (1997). *Self-efficacy: The exercise of control*. New York: Freeman.

Baranowski, T., Cullen, K., Nicklas, T., Thompson, D., & Baranowski, J. (2003). Are current health behavioral change models helpful in guiding prevention of weight gain efforts? *Obesity Research, 11*, 23–42.

Becker, M. H. (1974). The health belief model and personal health behavior. *Health Education Monographs, 2*, 324–473.

Bronfenbrenner, U. (1979). *The ecology of human development: Experiments by nature and design*. Cambridge, MA: Harvard University Press.

Champion, V., & Skinner, C. (2008). The health belief model. In K. Glanz, B. Rimer & K. Viswanath (Eds.), *Health behavior and health education: Theory, research, and practice* (4th ed., pp. 45–65). San Francisco: Jossey-Bass.

Consumer Health Informatics Research Resource (CHIRr). (2018). *Perceived Severity*. Retrieved from https://chirr.nlm.nih.gov/perceived-severity.php.

Cowdery, J. E., Wang, M. Q., Eddy, J. M., & Trucks, J. K. (1995). A theory driven health promotion program in a university setting. *Journal of Health Education, 26*, 248–250.

Crosby, R. A., Kegler, M. C., & DiClemente, R. J. (2002). Understanding and applying theory in health promotion practice and research. In R. J. DiClemente, R. A. Crosby, & M. C. Kegler (Eds.), *Emerging theories in health promotion practice and research: Strategies for improving public health* (pp. 1–15). San Francisco: Jossey-Bass.

D'Onofrio, C. N. (1992). Theory and the empowerment of health education practitioners. *Health Education Quarterly, 19*, 385–403.

Earp, J. A., & Ennett, S. T. (1991). Conceptual models for health education research and practice. *Health Education Research, 6*, 163–171.

Fiore, M. C., & Baker, T. B. (2009). Stealing a march in the 21st century: Accelerating progress in the 100-year war against tobacco addiction in the United States. *American Journal of Public Health, 99*, 1170–1175.

Glanz, K., & Rimer, B. K. (1995). *Theory at a glance: A guide for health promotion practice*. Washington, DC: National Cancer Institute.

Glanz, K., Rimer, B. K., & Viswanath, K. (2008). Theory, research, and practice in health behavior and health education. In K. Glanz, B. K. Rimer, & K. Viswanath (Eds.), *Health behavior and health education: Theory, research, and practice* (4th ed., pp. 23–40). San Francisco: Jossey-Bass.

Hochbaum, G. M. (1958). *Public participation in medical screening programs: A socio-psychological study*. Washington, DC: U.S. Department of Health, Education, and Welfare.

Hochbaum, G. M., Sorenson, J. R., & Lorig, K. (1992). Theory in health education practice. *Health Education Quarterly, 19*, 295–313.

Hruschka, D. J., & Hadley, C. (2008). A glossary of culture in epidemiology. *Journal of Epidemiology & Community Health, 62*, 947–951.

Janz, N. K. & Becker, M. H. (1984). The health belief model: A decade later. *Health Education Quarterly, 11*, 1–47.

Kirscht, J. P. (1974). The health belief model and illness behavior. *Health Education Monographs, 2*, 2387–2408.

McKenzie, J. F., Neiger, B. L., & Smeltzer, J. L. (2005). *Planning, implementing & evaluating health promotion programs*. San Francisco: Pearson Education.

McLeroy, K., Norton, B., Kegler, M., Burdine, J. N., & Sumaya, C. (2003). Community-based interventions. *American Journal of Public health, 93*, 529–533.

Poland, B. D., Green, L. W., & Rootman, I. (2000). *Settings for health promotion*. Thousand Oaks, CA: Sage.

Rimer, B. K. & Glanz, K. (2005). *Theory at a glance: A guide for health promotion practice* (2nd ed.). Washington, DC: National Cancer Institute.

Rogers, R. W. & Prentice-Dunn, S. (1997). *Protection motivation theory*. New York: Plenum.

Rosenstock, I. M. (1960). What research in motivation suggests for public health. *American Journal of Public Health, 50,* 295–302.

Rosenstock, I. M., Strecher, V. J., & Becker, M. H. (1988). Social learning theory and the health belief model. *Health Education Quarterly, 15,* 175–183.

Skinner, B. F. (1938). *The behavior of organisms.* Englewood Cliffs, NJ: Appleton-Century-Crofts.

Simons-Morton, B., McLeroy, K., & Wendel, M. (2012). *Behavior theory in health promotion practice and research.* Burlington, MA: Jones & Bartlett Learning.

Stokols, D. (1996). Translating social ecological theory into guidelines for community health promotion. *American Journal of Health Promotion, 10,* 282–298.

Tolman, E. C. (1932). *Purposive behavior in animals and men.* New York: Appleton-Century-Crofts.

Transportation Research Board, Institute of Medicine. (2005). *Does the built environment influence physical activity, examining the evidence.* Washington, DC: National Academies Press.

Watson, J. B. (1925). *Behaviorism.* New York: Norton.

Weinstein, N. D., Rothman, A. J., & Sutton, S. R. (1998). Stage theories of health behavior: Conceptual and methodological issues. *Health Psychology, 17,* 290–299.

Weinstein, N. D. & Sandman, P. M. (2002a). The precaution adoption process model and its application. In R. J. DiClemente, R. A. Crosby, & M. C. Kegler (Eds.), *Emerging theories in health promotion practice and research: Strategies for improving public health* (pp. 16–39). San Francisco: Jossey-Bass.

Weinstein, N. D. & Sandman, P. M. (2002b). The precaution adoption process model. In K. Glanz, B. K. Rimer, & F. M. Lewis (Eds.), *Health behavior and health education: Theory, research, and practice* (3rd ed., pp. 121–143). San Francisco: Jossey-Bass.

Witte, K. (1992). Putting the fear back into fear appeals: The extended parallel process model. *Communication Monographs, 59,* 329–349.

Chapter 4—Review Questions

1. Identify the differences between the following terms: attitudes, beliefs, knowledge, perceptions, and values.

2. Why is it important to utilize a theoretical framework when creating health promotion programs?

3. Describe the social ecological perspective. What does it imply regarding health behavior?

4. What is an intrapersonal model? Research and locate two research articles which utilize an intrapersonal model. Make sure to indicate which model was used in each article.

5. Identify the two basic assumptions the Health Belief Model was created upon. Are these assumptions still relevant now? Why or why not?

6. Review the Health Belief Model constructs. Provide an example survey question for each construct relating to breast cancer detection.

7. Cues to action is the hardest construct of the Health Belief Model to measure. Consider the past year and identify any cues to action which caused you to initiate a health behavior change.

8. What is self-efficacy and why is it so important to the Health Belief Model?

9. When utilizing the Health Belief Model as a theoretical framework, why is it important to use more than one question in a survey to measure each construct?

10. The inclusion of fear as an emotional construct for the Health Belief Model has been suggested by many researchers. Do you agree or disagree that fear is a strong predictor of health behavior? Why?

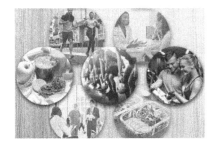

CHAPTER 5
Theory of Reasoned Action and Theory of Planned Behavior

This chapter covers material on two theories: the Theory of Reasoned Action (TRA) and the Theory of Planned Behavior (TPB). The TRA and the TPB focus on constructs concerned with individual motivational factors as determinants of the likelihood of performing a specific task or behavior. Both the TRA and the TPB have been successfully used to predict and explain a wide range of health behaviors, including smoking, alcohol use, substance use, physical activity, health care utilization, sun protection, breastfeeding, safer sexual behaviors, safety helmet use, and seat belt use. This chapter provides information on the history and origin of the TRA and the TPB, a description of the constructs which comprise each theory, and an example of the application of the TPB as it relates to safer sexual behaviors.

History of the Theory of Reasoned Action (TRA) and Theory of Planned Behavior (TPB)

Theory of Reasoned Action (TRA)

The **Theory of Reasoned Action** (TRA) was first developed to provide a better understanding of the relationships between beliefs, attitudes, intentions, and behaviors (Fishbein, 1967). The TRA was formulated in 1975 by psychologists Martin Fishbein and Icek Ajzen. It asserts that human social behavior is not controlled by unconscious motives; it is not thoughtless (Ajzen & Fishbein, 1980). The TRA states that people decide to engage or not engage in an action by careful consideration of its implications. Behavior is under volitional control, which means that it is a function of individual intention, or the degree an individual can exercise control, to perform a particular behavior. Individuals are more motivated to perform a behavior that will result in an outcome that is highly valued. When an individual does not believe that an act will lead to a specific outcome, or the outcome is not highly valued, the individual will be less motivated to perform the behavior.

Algebraically, the TRA can be represented as: $B \approx BI = w1AB + w2SN$

- B = behavior
- BI = behavioral intention
- AB = attitude toward behavior
- SN = subjective norm
- w1 & w2 = weights representing the importance of each term

The TRA works differently for different behaviors. For some behaviors, attitudes will have a greater ability to determine intentions; and for some behaviors, subjective norms will have a greater ability to determine intentions. Influencing factors may vary according to the target population, such as race, ethnicity, and age. The TRA posits that behavior is best predicted by behavioral intention, and intent is predicted by attitudes

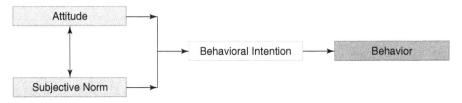

Figure 5.1. Theory of Reasoned Action (TRA).

toward the behavior and subjective norms toward the behavior (Simons-Morton, McLeroy, & Wendel, 2012). Figure 5.1 illustrates the relationships of the constructs which comprise the TRA.

The model has some limitations, including a significant risk of confounding between attitudes and norms, since attitudes can often be reframed as norms, and vice versa. A second limitation is the assumption that when we form an intention to act, we will be free to act without limitation. In practice, constraints such as limited ability, time, environmental or organizational limits, and unconscious habits will limit the freedom to act. The Theory of Planned Behavior (TPB) attempts to resolve this limitation (Eagly & Chaiken, 1993; Wade & Schneberger, 2012).

Theory of Planned Behavior (TPB)

The **Theory of Planned Behavior** (TPB) is one of the most influential theories for the prediction of social and health behaviors. This model is an extension of the TRA. In the TRA, behavior is under volitional control. The TPB goes beyond the TRA and addresses the problem of incomplete volitional control. According to the TPB, human behavior is guided by three kinds of considerations: (1) behavioral beliefs, (2) normative beliefs, and (3) control beliefs. Behavioral beliefs produce positive or negative attitudes toward the behavior. Normative beliefs result in perceived social pressure or subjective norms. Control beliefs lead to perceived behavioral control. In combination, attitude toward behavior, subjective norm, and perception of behavioral control lead to the formation of a behavioral intention. Given a sufficient degree of actual control over a particular behavior, individuals are expected to carry out their intended behavior. Intention is thus assumed to be the immediate antecedent of behavior. According to Ajzen (2002), the more favorable the attitude and subjective norm, and

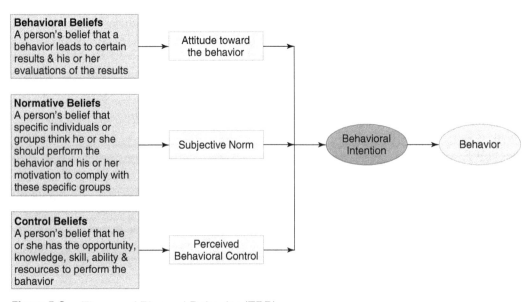

Figure 5.2. Theory of Planned Behavior (TPB).

the greater the perceived control, the stronger the person's intention should be to perform a particular behavior. Figure 5.2 illustrates the relationships of the constructs in the TPB.

Ajzen (1991) explicitly welcomed research which addresses the role of additional variables in the TPB, stating that "the theory of planned behavior is, in principle, open to the inclusion of additional predictors if it can be shown that they capture a significant portion of the variance in intention or behavior after the theory's current variables have been taken into account" (p. 199). Implications for further research include supporting the inclusion of an additional predictor in the theory. Emphasis should be placed upon expanding the current paradigm and explaining or accounting for new trends in behavior. It is important to note that the TPB may be applied in conjunction with other theories as well to design and deliver behavioral-change interventions. Thus, the TPB may complement the use of other theories and potentially improve behavioral-change research. The following section details the constructs of the TRA and the TPB.

Constructs of the TRA & TPB

Behavioral Beliefs

A **behavioral belief** is the subjective probability that the behavior will produce a given outcome. Behavioral beliefs link the behavior of interest to expected outcomes. Thus, it is assumed that these accessible beliefs determine one's *attitude* toward the behavior (Ajzen, 2002).

Attitudes

Attitudes toward a behavior are described as the individual's positive or negative feelings about performing the particular behavior. It is determined through an assessment of one's beliefs regarding the consequences arising from the behavior and an evaluation of the desirability of these consequences. "Favorable attitudes toward an object or action are positively associated with intent and action, while unfavorable attitudes toward an object or action are negatively associated with intent and action" (Simons-Morton et al., 2012, p.106). According to Ajzen (2002), the attitude toward a certain behavior is the degree to which the performance of the behavior is positively or negatively valued.

Normative Beliefs

Normative beliefs refer to the perceived behavioral expectations of important individuals or groups, such as a spouse, family members, teachers, coaches, and friends. It is assumed that normative beliefs (in combination with a person's motivation to comply with important people in their life who influence their behaviors), determine *subjective norms.*

Subjective Norms

Subjective norms are defined as the perceived social pressure to engage or not engage in a behavior. Subjective norms are also defined as "an individual's perception of whether people important to the individual think the behavior should be performed" (Ajzen, 1991). The contribution of the opinion of any given person of influential importance is weighted by the motivation an individual has to comply with the wishes of that referent.

Control Beliefs

Control beliefs deal with the perceived presence of factors that may facilitate or impede the performance of a behavior. It is assumed that control beliefs (in combination with the perceived power of each control factor) determine *perceived behavioral control.*

Perceived Behavioral Control

Perceived behavioral control refers to our perceptions of our ability to perform a given behavior. An individual's perception of control over behavioral performance is determined jointly by motivation (intention) and ability (perceived behavioral control). In other words, a person's perception of control over a particular behavior has a direct effect on the person's actual behavior (Ajzen, 1991). For example, if a college student demonstrates high perceived behavioral control relative to safer sexual practices, they are more likely to be confident in their ability to consistently use a condom.

Intention

The definition of **intention** is the cognitive representation of a person's readiness to perform a given behavior. Intention is considered to be the immediate antecedent of behavior. Intentions are based on attitudes, subjective norms, and perceived behavioral control.

Behavior Outcome

The **behavior outcome** is the resulting, observable response in a given situation with respect to a given target. According to the TPB, it is a function of compatible intentions and perceptions of behavioral control (Ajzen, 2002). The behavior outcome is the resulting health behavior change, such as quitting smoking, reducing stress, as well as consistent use of condoms and/or other contraceptives.

Application of the TPB

The TPB has been applied to explain a variety of health behaviors, including physical activity, smoking, drug use, HIV/STI prevention behaviors, mammography use, clinician provision of preventative health services, safety helmet use, seat belt use, as well as oral hygiene behaviors (Glanz, Rimer, & Lewis, 2002; Glanz, Rimer, & Viswanath, 2008; Rivis & Sheeran, 2003). In previous studies, intentions typically explained between 19% and 38% of the variance in behavior (Ajzen, 1991; Armitage & Conner, 2001). Attitudes and subjective norms (TRA) have accounted for 33%–50% of the variance in intentions. The addition of perceived behavioral control (TPB) typically increases the explained variance in intentions by 5%–12% (Ajzen, 1991; Sheeran & Taylor, 1997); and increases the variance explained in behavior by 2%–12% over and above intentions (Armitage & Conner, 2001).

When designing interventions, it is important to focus on factors underlying behaviors, such as attitudes or perceptions of norms that are changeable (Kasprzyk, Montano, & Fishbein, 1998). These findings may have the potential to drive the design of the intervention and health education messages.

A range of individual-level conceptual models have been proposed that differ in the specific social-cognitive factors and processes considered to be relevant to predict, understand, and change health-related behaviors (Fisher & Fisher, 2000; Wiggers, De Wit, Gras, Coutinho, & Van Den Hoek, 2003). According to Fisher and Fisher (2000), social-cognitive theories are increasingly being used to understand STIs and unintended pregnancy prevention practices, as well as to inform behavior change interventions in this field. The health belief model (HBM), presented in Chapter 4, proposed the earliest social cognitive account of health behavior.

As compared to the HBM, the TPB is viewed as a more complete theory of the proximal determinants of behavior. Any other factors that are external to the model are assumed to exert their influence on behavior only indirectly through the components of the TPB. These external factors include demographic characteristics, personality traits, as well as attitudinal and other individual difference variables. External factors include general health motivation, cues to action, and perceived health threat; which are key predictors of health behavior in the HBM (Wiggers et al., 2003). The evaluation of behavior relative to perceived benefits and costs as proposed by the HBM can be thought of as a reflection of beliefs underlying an individual's attitude toward the behavior. Self-efficacy considerations in the Health Belief Model are similar to the TPB's construct of perceived behavioral control (Ajzen, 1991).

TPB as Applied to Safer Sexual Behaviors

This section provides information on actions that promote responsible sexual behaviors through the application of the TPB. Responsible sexual behavior continues to be a major health issue for the nation, as the United States reports the highest rates of adolescent pregnancy and sexually transmitted infections (STIs) among industrialized nations. *Healthy People 2020* places responsible sexual behaviors as one of the leading health indicators (LHI) for the nation (CDC, 2018). Note that the title of this section refers to *safer* sexual behaviors, and not safe sexual behaviors. Individuals who participate in sexual behaviors with a partner (male or female) can increase their risk for unintended pregnancies and/or STIs; however, one can take precautions to minimize the likelihood of these possibilities.

In the past decade, there has been a great deal of research on the topic of factors associated with condom use, as well as the recognition of the need to develop theory-based behavioral interventions to increase condom use among those at most risk for STIs (youth ages 15–25). Researchers have focused on individual-difference factors in predicting and understanding a variety of health and social behaviors. Social-cognitive factors have been identified as the most important proximal determinants of behavior. These factors are generally focused on theory, research, and intervention practices due to the fact that they are open to change and can readily be targeted in a health promotion intervention (Wiggers et al., 2003).

In order to address the health issues of the nation, researchers apply models and theories to aid in the explanation of behavior. If researchers are better able to explain behaviors, then interventions may be developed to aid in the prevention of health-compromising behaviors. The TPB helps us to understand how we can change the behavior of people. The TPB can be used to predict safer sexual behaviors. For example, if a person has a positive attitude regarding contraceptives and perceives social pressure to use contraceptives, and also feels control over the ability to use contraceptives, that person will be more likely to attempt the behavior (Conner, Graham, & Moore, 1999). In other words, individuals are likely to intend to use condoms if they believe the behavior will lead to particular outcomes which they value, if they believe people whose views they value think they should carry out the behavior, and if they feel they have the necessary resources and opportunities to perform the behavior.

Behavioral interventions may be designed in order to change behavior and may be directed toward one or more of the TPB determinants: attitudes, subjective norms, or perceptions of behavioral control. According to the TPB, changes in these factors should produce changes in behavioral intentions, and given adequate control over the behavior, new intentions should be carried out under appropriate circumstances (Gollwitzer, 1999). Due to the fact that attitudes, subjective norms, and perceived behavioral control are assumed to be based on corresponding sets of beliefs, interventions must attempt to change the beliefs which guide the performance of a behavior. According to Ajzen (2002), one can determine the relative contributions of attitudes, subjective norms, and perceptions of behavioral control to the prediction of intentions as well as the relative contributions of intentions and perceptions of control to the prediction of behavior.

One can use a number of external variables to assist in the explanation of behaviors, such as age, sex, occupation, socioeconomic status, and education. An intervention or questionnaire could assess behavior beliefs (belief strength and outcome evaluations), normative beliefs (strength and motivation to comply), and control beliefs (strength and perceived power) (Ajzen, 2002). By measuring beliefs, one may gain insight into the underlying cognitive foundation, thus exploring why individuals hold certain attitudes, subjective norms, and perceptions of behavioral control. Beliefs provide a snapshot of the behavior's cognitive foundation within a given population at a given point in time.

An effective intervention method can be developed once it has been decided which beliefs the intervention will attempt to change. A number of interventions can incorporate the TPB; examples include educational programs, persuasive communications, ads, flyers, television and other social media messages (Ajzen, 2002). One must demonstrate that the intervention developed does in fact influence the beliefs it is designed to alter. Upon selecting a target for the behavioral intervention, an obvious consideration is whether or not there is much room for change in the target population. According to Ajzen and Fishbein (1980), if the formative research demonstrates there is room for change in two or all three predictors (i.e., attitudes, subjective norms, and perceived behavioral control), then it is possible to consider the relative weights in the prediction of intentions as well as behavior to target the intervention. In general, the greater the relative weight of a factor, the more likely it is that changing the factor will influence intentions and behavior.

For example, when applying the TPB to safer sexual behaviors, let's suppose that attitude toward condom use explains a great deal of the variance in behavioral intention. Subjective norms and perceptions of behavioral control contribute very little, and intentions account for most of the variance in behavior. Consequently, it would be most appropriate to direct the intervention at behavioral beliefs in an attempt to make attitudes toward the behavior more favorable, thus affecting intentions and the behavioral outcome.

Table 5.1. Constructs of the Theory of Planned Behavior (TPB) and Strategies for Health Educators.

Theory Component	Issue	Strategy/Goals for Health Educators
Behavioral Beliefs	Attitudes	Educational Interventions; Establish positive values and attitudes of behavior
Normative Beliefs	Subjective Norms	Peers as Role Models; Developing uniqueness in order to restrain social pressures
Control Beliefs	Perceived Control	Task/Performance Interventions; Enable individuals to perceive control over ability to perform tasks

Source: Penhollow, T. (2005). Responsible sexual behaviors: An application of the Theory of Planned Behavior (TPB). *Arkansas AHPERD Journal, 40,* 16–21.

In order to change attitudes, subjective norms, or perceived behavioral control, it is possible to attack either the strength of some of the relevant beliefs or their scale values. According to Ajzen (2002), only when the balance of beliefs in the total aggregate shifts in the desired direction can one expect a change in attitude toward a behavior. It is often easier to produce change by introducing information designed to lead to the formation of new beliefs than it is to change existing beliefs. It is thus important to ensure that the information provided is as accurate as possible.

Interventions directed at behavioral, normative, or control beliefs may succeed in producing corresponding changes in attitudes, subjective norms, and perceptions of behavioral control, and these changes may further influence intentions in the desired direction. The intervention may be less effective, however, if individuals are not capable of carrying out their newly formed intentions. It is important that the investigator form a strong link from intentions to behavior. The formation of plans detailing when, where, and how the desired behavior will be performed makes it easier for people to carry out their intended actions (Gollwitzer, 1999).

Interventions should be aimed at reducing the prevalence of health-risk behaviors as well as increasing health-enhancing behaviors. Descriptive norms in a number of studies have produced a larger regression coefficient in the prediction of intention compared with subjective norms (Rivis & Sheeran, 2003; Wiggers et al., 2003). Thus observing the behavior of others may be of greater importance in health-related decision-making than social pressure from others. Table 5.1 illustrates components of the TPB and provides examples of potential intervention strategies for health educators.

The TPB can be used to plan a health promotion intervention aimed at increasing awareness and utilization of condoms among college students. For example, health education specialists may use a survey to assess variables which measure the TPB constructs. A number of the example questions provided in Table 5.2 have been used in previous research to address condom use among college students (Bennett & Bozionelos, 2000; Broaddus, Schmiege, & Bryan, 2011; Penhollow, Young, & Bailey, 2007; Penhollow, Young, & Denny, 2005; Reid & Aiken, 2011; Simons-Morton et al., 2012; Young, Penhollow, & Bailey, 2010). Table 5.2 presents definitions and examples of the TPB constructs as applied to safer sexual behaviors.

The example questions provided in Table 5.2 can be used in a survey instrument designed to assess the effectiveness of a health promotion intervention aimed at condom use among college students. The identical questionnaire should be given before the educational intervention and immediately after the health promotion intervention. If the survey is simply given before the intervention and not after the intervention, or vice versa, one cannot assess the impact the intervention had on the participants. Additionally, a design which includes a control group is imperative in order to determine whether any change or lack of change among intervention participants can be directly attributed to the educational intervention. Assessing the effectiveness of a health promotion program is vital to the success and longevity of the program. After evaluation, if a program does not prove to be successful, (lead to positive health behavior change), steps need to be taken to considerably alter the health promotion intervention.

Table 5.2.   Definitions and Examples of the TPB as Applied to Safer Sexual Behaviors.

- **Behavioral Beliefs**—Beliefs about the consequences of a behavior.
  - *Example question*: Consistent condom use is an effective way to prevent unintended pregnancy and STIs. (Strongly Agree, Agree, Disagree, Strongly Disagree)
  - **Attitudes Toward Behavior**—Positive or negative evaluation of performing a particular behavior.
    - *Example question*: Condom use does not impede my sexual satisfaction. (Strongly Agree, Agree, Disagree, Strongly Disagree)
- **Normative Beliefs**—Perception about a behavior as influenced by the judgment of significant others.
  - *Example question*: Most of my friends use condoms when they have sex. (Strongly Agree, Agree, Disagree, Strongly Disagree)
  - **Subjective Norms**—Beliefs about the extent to which significant others approve or disapprove of a particular behavior.
    - *Example question*: My friends and family would approve of my use of condoms as a way to protect myself. (Strongly Agree, Agree, Disagree, Strongly Disagree)
- **Control Beliefs**—Evaluation of one's ability to engage in the intended behavior.
  - *Example question*: I am capable of using condoms every time I participate in sexual intercourse. (Strongly Agree, Agree, Disagree, Strongly Disagree)
  - **Perceived Behavioral Control**— Evaluation of the factors that may impede the performance of a particular behavior.
    - *Example question*: I do not believe any barriers exist in using condoms when I participate in sexual intercourse. (Strongly Agree, Agree, Disagree, Strongly Disagree)
- **Intention**—Evaluation of the readiness to perform a particular behavior.
  - *Example question*: I am likely to use condoms when I participate in sexual intercourse. (Strongly Agree, Agree, Disagree, Strongly Disagree)
  - **Behavioral Outcome**—The resulting, observable action in response to a given situation.
    - *Example question*: How often did you use a condom when engaging in sexual intercourse in the past 30 days? (Always, Most of the time, Some of the time, Never)

Summary

This chapter provided information on two intrapersonal-level theories: the Theory of Reasoned Action (TRA) and the Theory of Planned Behavior (TPB). Both the TRA and the TPB have been used as theoretical frameworks for studying and explaining many types of health behavior. The TRA focuses on cognitive factors (attitudes and subjective norms) that determine motivation of behavior (intention). It has been useful in explaining behavior under volitional control. The TPB extends the TRA by adding perceived behavioral control, which is concerned with facilitating or constraining conditions which affect intention and behavior. This is essential for behaviors over which an individual has less perceived volitional control. Volitional control is similar to the construct of self-efficacy. In other words, having or perceiving control and/or being confident to perform a particular health behavior. This chapter also provided content on the application of the TPB as applied to safer sexual behaviors.

References

Ajzen, I. (1991). The theory of planned behavior (TPB). *Organizational Behavior and Human Decision Processes, 50*, 179–211.

Ajzen, I. (2002). *The theory of planned behavior (TPB).* Retrieved from http://www-unix.oit.umass.edu/~aizen/tpb.html.

Ajzen, I., & Fishbein, M. (1980). *Understanding attitudes and predicting social behavior.* Englewood Cliffs, NJ: Prentice-Hall.

Armitage, C. J., & Conner, M. (2001). Efficacy of the theory of planned behavior: A meta-analytic review. *British Journal of Social Psychology, 40*, 471–499.

Bennett, P., & Bozionelos, G. (2000). The theory of planned behaviour as predictor of condom use: A narrative review. *Psychology, Health & Medicine, 5*, 307–327.

Broaddus, M., Schmiege, S., & Bryan, A. (2011). An expanded model of the temporal stability of condom use intentions: Gender-specific predictors among high-risk adolescents. *Annals of Behavioral Medicine, 42*, 99–110.

Centers for Disease Control and Prevention. (2018). *Healthy People 2020.* Retrieved from https://www.healthypeople.gov.

Conner, M., Graham, S., & Moore, B. (1999). Alcohol and intentions to use condoms: Applying the theory of planned behavior. *Psychology & Health, 14*, 795–812.

Eagly, A. H., & Chaiken, S. (1993). *The psychology of attitudes.* Fort Worth, TX: Harcourt Brace Jovanovich College Publishers.

Fishbein, M. (1967). *Readings in attitude theory and measurement.* New York: Wiley.

Fishbein, M., & Ajzen, I. (1975). *Belief, attitude, intention, and behavior: An introduction to theory and research.* Reading, MA: Addison-Wesley.

Fisher, J. D., & Fisher, W. A. (2000). Theoretical approaches to individual-level change in HIV risk behavior. In *Handbook of HIV Prevention* (pp. 3–55). New York: Plenum.

Glanz, K., Rimer, B. K., & Lewis, F. M. (2002). *Health behavior and health education: Theory, research, and practice* (3rd ed.). San Francisco: John Wiley.

Glanz, K., Rimer, B. K., & Viswanath, K. (2008). *Health behavior and health education: Theory, research, and practice* (4th ed.). San Francisco: John Wiley.

Gollwitzer, P. M. (1999). Implementation intentions: Strong effects of simple plans. *American Psychologist, 54*, 493–503.

Kasprzyk, D., Montano, D. E., & Fishbein, M. (1998). Application of an integrated behavioral model to predict condom use: A prospective study among high HIV risk groups. *Journal of Applied Social Psychology, 28*, 1557–1583.

Penhollow, T. (2005). Responsible sexual behaviors: An application of the Theory of Planned Behavior (TPB). *Arkansas AHPERD Journal, 40*, 16–21.

Penhollow, T., Young, M., & Bailey, W. (2007). Relationship between religiosity and hooking up behavior. *American Journal of Health Education, 38*, 338–345.

Penhollow, T., Young, M., & Denny, G. (2005). Impact of religiosity on the sexual behaviors of college students. *American Journal of Health Education, 36*, 75–83.

Reid, A., & Aiken, L. (2011). Integration of five health behaviour models: Common strengths and unique contributions to understanding condom use. *Psychology & Health, 26*, 1499–1520.

Rivis, A., & Sheeran, P. (2003). Descriptive norms as an additional predictor in the Theory of Planned Behavior: A meta-analysis. *Current Psychology: Developmental, Learning, Personality, Social, 22*, 218–233.

Sheeran, P., & Taylor, S. (1997). Predicting intentions to use condoms: Meta-analysis and comparison of theories of reasoned action and planned behavior. *Journal of Applied Social Psychology, 29*, 1624–1675.

Simons-Morton, B., McLeroy, K., & Wendel, M. (2012). *Behavior theory in health promotion practice and research*. Burlington, MA: Jones & Bartlett.

Wade, M., & Schneberger, S. (2012). *Theories used in IS research: Theory of Reasoned Action*. York University. Retrieved from http://www.istheory.yorku.ca/theoryofreasonedaction.htm.

Wiggers, L. C. W., De Wit, J. B. F., Gras, M. J., Coutinho, R. A., & Van Den Hoek, A. (2003). Risk behavior and social-cognitive determinants of condom use among ethnic minority communities in Amsterdam. *AIDS Education and Prevention, 15*, 430–447.

Young, M., Penhollow, T., & Bailey, W. (2010). Hooking-up and condom provision: Is there a double standard? *American Journal of Health Studies, 25*, 156–164.

Chapter 5—Review Questions

1. Compare and contrast the TRA and the TPB. How do these theories differ regarding volitional control?

2. Identify and describe the two main determinants of behavior that lead to intention according to the TRA.

3. Identify and describe the three main determinants of behavior that lead to intention according to the TPB.

4. Review the constructs of the TPB. Which construct accounts for peer pressure?

5. Behavioral outcomes result from congruency between intention and perceived behavioral control. Provide an example statement for intention and perceived behavioral control which would lead to the behavioral outcome of exercising.

6. When a health education specialist is planning an intervention using the TRA or TPB, which two factors should be the central focus? Why?

7. Identify five external factors which would indirectly influence behavior through the constructs of the TPB.

8. Recall the Health Belief Model (HBM). The HBM and the TPB contain at least one construct which is similar. Identify and define at least one similar construct from each model/theory.

9. Provide an example survey question for each construct of the TPB as related to seat belt use.

10. Refer to Table 5.1. What additional strategies or goals could be used by health educators to address binge drinking among college students?

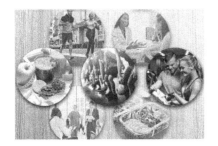

CHAPTER 6
The Transtheoretical Model and Stages of Change

This chapter provides a summary of the Transtheoretical Model (TTM). As previously stated in Chapter 4, the TTM is one of many stage theories. The TTM categorizes people into stages according to their preparedness, or lack of preparedness, to modify or change a certain behavior. Originally, the TTM was used in smoking-cessation interventions; however, its application has expanded to encompass topics such as mental health, substance abuse, eating disorders, and cancer prevention. This chapter will discuss the history of the TTM, explain the stages of change and the processes of change, and provide an example application of the TTM within health education research.

History of the Transtheoretical Model (TTM)

"The **Transtheoretical Model** is an integrative framework for understanding how individuals and populations progress toward adopting and maintaining health behavior change for optimal health" (Prochaska, Johnson, & Lee, 1998). The TTM emerged from various psychotherapy and behavior-change studies. In 1979, Prochaska developed the TTM after comparatively analyzing 18 therapy systems and conducting 300 critical reviews on therapy-outcome studies (Prochaska, 1979). The TTM is a combination of many popular psychotherapy interventions, including psychological approaches from Freud, Skinner, and Rogers, and this is how the name "transtheoretical" originated.

The TTM is an intentional behavior change model which describes the stages of change individuals move through and the mechanisms they use to help modify or change their health behavior. In other words, the TTM addresses *how* an individual makes a behavioral modification rather than *why*. In Chapter 4, the Health Belief Model (HMB) constructs of perceived susceptibility and perceived severity addressed *why* an individual would make a behavior change. The TTM addresses *how* an individual successfully modifies behavior and maintains the behavior change long-term.

Similar to most health behavior models or theories, the TTM is based upon assumptions regarding the nature of behavior change. It is important for health educators to understand these core assumptions when deciding which behavior change theory is the best fit for their intervention. Assumptions of the TTM include (Prochaska, Redding, & Evers, 2008):

- No single theory can account for all complexities of behavioral change. A more comprehensive model is most likely to emerge from integration across major theories.
- Behavior change is a process that unfolds over time through a sequence of stages.
- Stages are both stable and open to change, just as chronic behavioral risk factors are stable and open to change.
- The majority of at-risk populations are not prepared for action and will not be served effectively by traditional action-oriented behavior change programs.
- Specific processes and principles of change should be emphasized at specific stages to maximize efficacy.

Stages of Change

The TTM describes behavior change as a process which occurs over time. The stages of change integrate the component of time in a linear model; however, individuals may move freely between stages as their preparedness to change either increases or decreases. Table 6.1 provides the typical timeframe during which an individual experiences the different stages. Since each stage presents individuals with different challenges, stage-matched interventions have been utilized to transition individuals from one stage to the next. The concept of stage-matched interventions will be discussed in more detail later in the chapter. There are six stages of change which compose the TTM: (1) precontemplation, (2) contemplation, (3) preparation, (4) action, (5) maintenance, and (6) termination. Figure 6.1 depicts the stages of change as a pyramid which individuals must climb in order to achieve long-term change.

Precontemplation

In the **precontemplation** stage, individuals are not even thinking about changing, and do not intend to participate in behavioral change in the near future, typically measured as the next six months. They may be in this stage because they are unaware of any need for a behavioral change or because they attempted to change in the past and have relapsed and are too discouraged to attempt change again. These individuals are typically not ready for health promotion programs and may resist interventions.

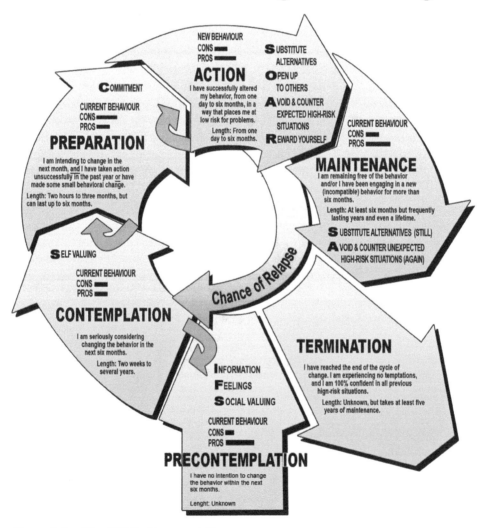

Figure 6.1. The TTM's Stages of Change.

Table 6.1.   Stages of Change Timeframe.

Precontemplation	No intention to change in the next six months
Contemplation	Intention to change in the next six months
Preparation	Intention to change within the next month
Action	Observable change has occurred during the last six months
Maintenance	Observable change has occurred for six months to five years or longer
Termination	Observable change has occurred for more then six years with no temptation to relapse

From *Handbook of Health Promotion and Disease Prevention*, Table 1.1, Page 42, by Raczynski and DiClemente. Copyright © 1999 Kluwer Academic / Plenum Publishers. With kind permission from Springer Science+Business Media B.V.

Contemplation

Individuals in the **contemplation** stage intend to participate in a behavior change within the next six months. Contemplators are more aware of the necessity to change in comparison to precontemplators. It is at this stage that individuals weigh both the pros and cons of behavior change, which is known as **decisional balance**. Contemplation is similar to the constructs of perceived benefits and perceived barriers found in the HBM. Contemplating the pros and cons of a behavior change can leave an individual in the contemplation stage for a prolonged period of time which is considered chronic contemplation.

Preparation

In the **preparation stage**, an individual intends to participate in behavior change within the next month. During this stage an individual takes steps to prepare for the behavior change. Preparations may include joining a gym, meeting with a nutritionist, consulting a physician, or signing up for a health education course. Individuals in the preparation stage are excellent candidates for action-based interventions since they have decided to make a behavior change and are actively seeking consultation or assistance.

Action

In the **action** stage, individuals have made observable behavior modifications within the last six months. However, not all behavior modifications are considered action; therefore, it is imperative to set behavioral criteria in order to distinguish the difference between action and preparation. For example, an individual who gradually decreases the number of cigarettes smoked each day is considered to be in the preparation stage. The individual enters the action stage only by completely giving up cigarette smoking.

Maintenance

Individuals in the **maintenance** stage are working to prevent relapse. Typically, they have a decreased temptation to relapse and do not need to work as hard as individuals in the action stage. Depending upon the individual and the behavior modification, the maintenance stage can last from six months to five years or longer.

Termination

In the **termination** stage, individuals are 100% free from temptation and relapse. No matter what the circumstances, individuals who have reached the termination stage will not go back to the unhealthy behavior. Those who have progressed to the termination stage have been in the maintenance stage for at least five years. An adult who practices consistent seat belt use is an example of an individual in the termination stage—he or she automatically puts on a seat belt whenever in a vehicle. Other behavior modifications which are not automatic, such as exercise, diet, and substance cessation, may become lifetime maintenance, since relapse is prevalent among those behaviors. Research on the termination stage is sparse in comparison to the other stages of change in the Transtheoretical Model.

While the stages of change present a linear model, behavior change does not always occur in a forward, linear motion for every individual. As individuals undertake behavior change, they may relapse to a previous stage. It is critical to understand that it may take multiple attempts at behavior change for some individuals to reach the maintenance or termination stage. Cycling and recycling through the stages of change is an inherent characteristic of behavior change and should be considered when creating behavior change interventions. Remobilizing such individuals and getting them back on track to achieve behavior change is no small task for an intervention. To maximize intervention efforts, participants should be encouraged to focus on what they have learned from their experience of relapse so they can prepare for their next behavior change effort.

Processes of Change

"**Processes of change** are the covert and overt activities people use to progress through stages" (Prochaska et al., 2008). Processes are the actual mechanisms through which individuals achieve the desired behavior modification. These are important guides for health educators to utilize while developing interventions, because they provide the framework with which to design a behavior change intervention (DiClemente, Redding, Crosby, & Salazar, 2013). Interventions which are aimed at modifying an individual's attitudes, emotions, or behaviors should incorporate at least one process of change strategy. Once the intervention is implemented, the health educator should utilize these processes to help the program participants progress through the stages of change with the ultimate goal of lifetime behavior change. Figure 6.2 illustrates how the processes of change are correlated to the stages of change. Ten processes of change have been substantiated by empirical support (Table 6.2): (1) consciousness raising, (2) dramatic relief, (3) self-reevaluation, (4) environmental reevaluation, (5) self-liberation, (6) helping relationships, (7) counterconditioning, (8) contingency management, (9) stimulus control, and (10) social liberation.

Consciousness Raising

Consciousness raising involves increasing awareness regarding the causes, consequences, and treatments for a negative health behavior. For example, unprotected, prolonged exposure to sunlight increases the risk for developing skin cancer; however, using sunscreen, which protects the skin from UVA/UVB rays, decreases the chances of developing skin cancer. Interventions can incorporate consciousness raising by providing basic health information to the program participants in the form of pamphlets, brochures, media service announcements, classroom education and/or providing sunscreen products to promote the use of sun protection.

Dramatic Relief

Dramatic relief produces an increase in emotional expression—specifically anxiety and fear; however, such expressions can be dispelled if appropriate action is taken. For example, seeing pictures of blackened and damaged lungs may produce an emotional response within a smoker. Media campaigns, personal testimonials, and pictures can be utilized during interventions to produce an affective reaction within the program participants.

Stages of Change -->						
Processes						
Precontemplation	**Contemplation**	**Preparation**	**Action**	**Maintenance**	**Termination**
Consciousness raising					
Dramatic relief					
Environmental reevaluation					
	Self-reevaluation				
		Self-liberation			
		Contingency management			
		Helping relationships			
		Counterconditioning			
		Stimulus control			
		Social liberation			

Figure 6.2.   Processes of Change for Progress Through the Stages of Change.

Table 6.2. Processes of Change and Sample Intervention Strategies

Consciousness raising	Increasing information about the healthy behavior change and awareness of one's risks: media campaigns, feedback, confrontations
Dramatic relief	Experiencing and expressing emotions associated with engaging in un-healthy behaviors: role playing, mass media messages, personal testimonies
Self-reevaluation	Realizing how one thinks and feels about oneself (i.e., self-image) with regard to engaging in an unhealthy behavior and how one's self-image might change if the behavior were to be changed: values clarification, imagery, exposure to healthy role models
Environmental reevaluation	Assessing how one's behavior may negatively impact others in her or his personal-social environment, or affect the physical environment: empathy training, documentaries, couple-family system interventions
Self-liberation	Choosing and firmly committing to change: go "public" with one's decision to change, set a "quit," or "start" date, empowerment
Helping relationships	Having someone to talk to, share feelings with, and get feedback from regarding the healthy behavior change: Increasing social support, rapport building, therapeutic alliances
Counterconditioning	Learning new healthy behaviors to substitute for old unhealthy ones: relaxation exercises, assertiveness training, increasing positive "self-talk"
Contingency management	Rewarding oneself or being rewarded by others for making a healthy change: contingency contracts, overt and covert reinforcements
Stimulus control	Avoiding people, places, or situations that might trigger unhealthy behavior and adding cues to trigger healthy behavior: avoidance techniques, restructuring one's environment (e.g., removing alcohol or fatty foods; carrying condoms), posting reminders to engage in healthy behaviors (e.g., taking prescribed medications)
Social liberation	Realizing changes in social norms with regard to certain health behaviors: advocacy, public policy changes (e.g., smoke-free malls, restaurants, schools)

Self-Reevaluation

Self-reevaluation is an individual's own assessment of his or her self-image as it reflects a certain behavior. More specifically, it encompasses both cognitive and emotional assessments by the individual. For example, an obese individual would visualize going through life as a sedentary person, but would also visualize what life might be as a fit and energetic person.

Environmental Reevaluation

Environmental reevaluation is a cognitive and affective assessment of how an individual's behavior, or lack of behavior, affects their social environment. For example, a smoker assesses the impact of secondhand smoke on other people in the surrounding area. This process may also include an increased awareness of being a role model (positive or negative). For example, if a teenager observes a parent smoking cigarettes, the teenager may believe smoking is not a harmful behavior and model after the parent's behavior. Interventions which encourage receiving feedback from other family members, friends, teachers, and coaches regarding the impact of the negative health behavior may spark a reevaluation within the program participant.

Self-Liberation

Self-liberation is the belief that individuals can make a behavioral change and the commitment they have to that belief. In other words, if you announce to family, friends, and co-workers that you will start eating properly and exercising, you may feel more empowered to actually make the desired behavior change. Encouraging intervention participants to share the goals they have set with family and friends may increase their willpower to reach the desired behavior change. On the other hand, self-liberation may mean making a promise to yourself, as to not let others negatively influence or discourage your decisions, and then letting family and friends notice your health behavior change.

Helping Relationships

Helping relationships encompass caring, trust, and acceptance to support an individual through the desired behavior change. Having the support of a helping relationship will greatly influence an individual's progress through the stages of change. For example, if an individual decides to start exercising, having an exercise buddy can increase the individual's willingness to exercise. Being committed to another person or group can increase the likelihood of participation in a healthy behavior. Interventions which use trust-building exercises and the buddy system provide program participants with much-needed social support during their behavior change.

Counterconditioning

Counterconditioning is the substitution of a positive health behavior for a negative health behavior. For example, instead of smoking cigarettes to ease stress, an individual may take a yoga class or practice meditation to decrease stress. Instead of coming home from work or school and having a drink, an individual may substitute that behavior with going for a walk. Typically, counterconditioning requires learning and/or practicing a new health behavior.

Contingency Management

Contingency management provides a reward-and-punishment system depending upon the direction an individual takes during the behavior change. Typically, rewards are better than punishments at impacting behavioral change. For example, an individual trying to quit smoking could be rewarded with a desirable item of choice at the end of the week or the end of the month with all of the money saved by not smoking. Interventions which incorporate incentives may increase the chance of program participants reaching their desired behavior change.

Stimulus Control

Stimulus control removes cues to negative health behaviors and adds new cues related to the desired behavior change. For example, some people may be less tempted to smoke a cigarette while driving if they do not have cigarettes in their car. People are also less likely to smoke if they spend their time with people who do not participate in that behavior. Many people may exercise more if they keep workout apparel in their car, at work, or at the gym instead of having to go home first. Avoidance and changing social environments will reduce the risk of relapsing to the undesired behavior.

Social Liberation

Social liberation utilizes social opportunities to reinforce positive health behaviors. For example, the movement to eliminate trans fats from foods has largely promoted better nutrition. Policies which provide schoolchildren with healthful foods at lunch are continually advocating positive behavior change. Availability of free contraceptives and free HIV/AIDS testing promote positive health behaviors as well.

Additional TTM Constructs

In addition to the stages of change and processes of change, the TTM is comprised of two other key constructs: decisional balance and self-efficacy. Decisional balance was introduced earlier in this chapter as weighing the pros and cons of behavior change, especially during the contemplation stage. **Self-efficacy** was defined earlier in the text (see Chapter 4) as an individual's confidence in having the ability to perform a desired behavior (Bandura, 1997).

Decisional Balance

Decisional balance was derived from studies relating to decision-making (Janis & Mann, 1977). Originally, the TTM adopted four categories of pros and four categories of cons created by Janis and Mann. However, after many studies tried to reproduce these eight factors, a much simpler two-factor structure of the pros and cons of behavior change was found (Prochaska et al., 2008).

Decisional balance and its correlation with the stages of change have been substantiated empirically through meta-analysis. It was through meta-analysis that both the Strong Principle and the Weak Principle were found. The **Strong Principle** posits that the pros of health behavior change must increase by one standard deviation (SD) from the precontemplation stage to the action stage (Prochaska, 1994). The **Weak Principle** posits that the cons of the health behavior change must decrease by one-half SD from the precontemplation stage to the action stage (Hall & Rossi, 2008). These principles indicate that the pros of changing must increase twice as much as the cons of changing must decrease in order for behavior change to occur. Therefore, it may be beneficial for interventions to emphasize the benefits of behavior change in order to make the barriers to behavior change smaller. For example, if a sedentary individual can only list five or six benefits of exercise and two or three barriers to exercise, the barriers may outweigh the benefits. However, if the sedentary individual could list 10 benefits of exercising, the three barriers originally listed would be small in comparison to the benefits. Additionally, these principles provide evidence which suggests there is a clear point when an individual favors the pros when weighing the pros and cons of behavior change. This is an important finding because an individual who reaches that point is able to move to the next stage of change.

Self-Efficacy

The construct of self-efficacy was conceptualized by Albert Bandura during his behavior therapy work (Bandura, 1986). Self-efficacy as a construct of the TTM encompasses two components: confidence and temptation (DiClemente & Prochaska, 1982; Velicer, DiClemente, Rossi, & Prochaska, 1990). **Confidence** refers to an individual's perception of having the ability to cope with high-risk situations without relapsing to the negative health behavior. **Temptation** addresses the intense urges experienced during high-risk situations. In situations where confidence is low and temptation is high, an individual is at an increased risk for relapse. When confidence is high and temptation is low, an individual is at low risk for relapse. High confidence and low temptation provide the optimal environment for a successful behavior change.

Application of the TTM

Initially, the TTM was created for the purpose of smoking-cessation interventions; however, it has been applied to various other health interventions. The number of diverse studies which adopted the TTM as a theoretical framework for behavior change has provided robust empirical support for the TTM constructs (Noar, Benac, & Harris, 2007). Interventions such as stage-matched peer advisers (Cabral et al., 1996), motivational interviewing (DiClemente & Velasquez, 2002), and stage-matched material contain elements of the TTM.

When implementing a stage-matched intervention, it is important for health educators to determine in which stage participants belong. Staging is a process which establishes an individual's readiness for behavior change. This is a crucial first step, because once an individual is "staged," the proper intervention strategies, or processes of change, can be utilized in order to assist in the individual's progress to the next stage. For example, Duane and Brett both smoke a pack of cigarettes a day but want to quit smoking. Even though they both smoke the same number of cigarettes, it is still necessary to determine their readiness to quit and "stage" them in the proper stage of change. Duane has attempted to quit smoking multiple times before, but has not been successful in quitting for good. On the other hand, Brett has never attempted to quit smoking, but he has considered quitting before. In this example, Duane would be placed in the preparation stage because he has already made multiple attempts to quit, whereas, Brett would be placed in the contemplation stage because he has only considered or thought about quitting smoking. Based upon their stage placement, Duane and Brett would be provided with different intervention strategies in order to move them to the next stage.

Following is an example of how the TTM was applied to promote contraceptive and condom use. Project PROTECT was a computer-delivered, TTM-tailored feedback system designed to promote contraceptive and condom use among at-risk young women. Project PROTECT screened, recruited, and randomized young women, using a baseline measurement, into either a standard-care group or a TTM intervention group (Peipert et al., 2007). All study participants (N = 542) received a baseline medical examination to ensure they did not have a sexually transmitted infection (STI). After the baseline measurement, STI, contraceptive use, and unintentional pregnancies were tracked for the next 24 months. The women in the standard-care group received a medical evaluation, treatment, and one computerized session with generic information regarding contraceptive and condom use. However, the women in the TTM intervention group received a medical evaluation, treatment, and up to three computerized sessions which were tailored to their readiness to use contraceptives and condoms.

The TTM computerized sessions were delivered over a 30-minute time span and included sections on both contraceptive and condom use. The sessions started with tailored feedback relating to the participant's stages of contraceptive use, pros and cons of contraceptive use, and efficacy for contraceptive use. The second section of the TTM intervention included more detailed feedback regarding condom use. The condom-use section included the targeting stages of condom use in general, stages of condom use for main partner(s), stages of condom use for other partner(s), pros and cons of condom use, efficacy of condom use, and processes of condom use (Redding, Morokoff, Rossi, & Meier, 2008). Data were collected in order to decide which processes of change to provide feedback for in each stage of condom use. At the completion of the study, the TTM intervention group was 70% more likely to use both contraceptives and condoms, as compared to the standard-care group. Therefore, the participants who received the stage-matched intervention increased their health protective behaviors more than the participants who received the generic intervention. However, there were no statistically significant differences between the two groups regarding the incidence of STIs and unintended pregnancies (Peipert et al., 2008).

Summary

The TTM is an intentional behavior change model which assesses an individual's readiness to modify behavior. The TTM comprises stages of change, which range from having no intention to modify behavior to successfully modifying the behavior and being free from behavioral relapse. The six stages of change include: (1) precontemplation, (2) contemplation, (3) preparation, (4) action, (5) maintenance, and (6) termination. In order for an individual to progress through the stages of change, there are necessary mechanisms called processes of change which the individual should utilize. There are 10 processes of change which have multiple empirical support and were discussed in this chapter. Additionally, the TTM has two other constructs which make behavior change possible: decisional balance and self-efficacy. Each of these constructs was examined in detail relating to the TTM. While the TTM was initially used in smoking-cessation interventions, the chapter presented the TTM as applied to an intervention which encouraged contraceptive and condom use among young women.

References

Bandura, A. (1986). *Social foundations of thought & action: A social cognitive theory.* Upper Saddle River, NJ: Prentice Hall.

Bandura, A. (1997). *Self-efficacy: The exercise of control.* New York: Freeman.

Cabral, R. J., Galavotti, C., Gargiullo, P. M., Armstrong, K., Cohen, A., Geilen, A. C., & Watkinson, L. (1996). Paraprofessional delivery of a theory-based HIV prevention counseling intervention for women. *Public Health Reports, 3,* 75–82.

DiClemente, C. C., & Prochaska, J. O. (1982). Self-changing and therapy change of smoking behavior: A comparison of processes of change in cessation and maintenance. *Addictive Behavior, 7,* 133–142.

DiClemente, C. C., & Velasquez, M. W. (2002). Motivational interviewing and the stages of change. In W. R. Miller & S. Rollnick (Eds.), *Motivational interviewing: Preparing people for change* (2nd ed., pp. 217–250). New York: Guilford Press.

DiClemente, R. J., Redding, C. A., Crosby, R. A., & Salazar, L. F. (2013). Stage models for health promotion. In R. J. DiClemente, L. F. Salazar, & R. A. Crosby (Eds.), *Health behavior theory for public health: Principles, foundations, and applications* (pp. 105–129). Burlington, MA: Jones & Bartlett Learning.

Hall, K. L., & Rossi, J. S. (2008). Meta-analytic examination of the strong and weak principles across 48 health behaviors. *Preventative Medicine, 46,* 266–274.

Janis, I. L., & Mann, L. (1977). *Decision making: A psychological analysis of conflict, choice, and commitment.* New York: Free Press.

Noar, S. M., Benac, C., & Harris, M. (2007). Does tailoring matter? Meta-analytical review of tailored print health behavior change interventions. *Psychological Bulletin, 133,* 673–693.

Peirpet, J. F., Redding, C. A., Blume, J., Allsworth, J., Ianucillo, K., Lozowski, F., & Rossi, J. S. (2007). Design of a stage-matched intervention trial to increase dual method contraceptive use (Project PROTECT). *Contemporary Clinical Trials, 28,* 626–637.

Peirpet, J. F., Redding, C. A., Blume, J., Allsworth, J., Matteson, K., Lozowski, F., & Rossi, J. S. (2008). Tailored intervention trial to increase dual methods: A randomized trial to reduce unintended pregnancies and sexually transmitted infections. *American Journal of Obstetrics & Gynecology, 198,* 630e1–630e8.

Prochaska, J. O. (1979). *Systems of psychotherapy: A transtheoretical analysis.* Homewood, IL: Dorsey Press.

Prochaska, J. O. (1994). Common principles for progression from precontemplation to action based on twelve problem behaviors. *Health Psychology, 13,* 47–51.

Prochaska, J. O., Johnson, S., & Lee, P. (1998). The transtheoretical model of behavior change. In S. A. Shumaker, E. B. Schron, J. K. Ockene, & W. L. McBee (Eds.), *The handbook of health behavior change* (2nd ed., pp. 59–84). New York: Springer.

Prochaska, J. O., Redding, C. A., & Evers, K. E. (2008). The transtheoretical model and stages of change. In K. Glanz, B. K. Rimer, & K. Viswanath (Eds.), *Health behavior and health education: Theory, research, and practice* (4th ed., pp. 97–121). San Francisco: Jossey-Bass.

Redding, C. A., Morokoff, P. J., Rossi, J. S., & Meier, K. S. (2008). One session intervention for at-risk women and men. In T. Edgar, S. Noar, & V. Friemuth (Eds.), *Communication perspectives on HIV/AIDS for the 21st century* (pp. 423–428). Mahwah, NJ: Lawrence Erlbaum.

Velicer, W. R., DiClemente, C. C., Rossi, J. S., & Prochaska, J. O. (1990). Relapse situations and self-efficacy: An integrative model. *Addictive Behaviors, 15,* 271–283.

Chapter 6—Review Questions

1. Explain what a stage theory is and why the Transtheoretical Model (TTM) is considered to be a stage theory.

2. Identify and describe the stages of change which compose the TTM.

3. What is decisional balance and in which stage of change can it be located?

4. Would individuals in the precontemplation stage be ready to join an intervention program? Why or why not?

5. What are the processes of change? Why are they so important in the practice of health education?

6. Define social liberation. Provide two examples of social liberation within your community.

7. Consider the stages of change and the processes of change. How do they work together within an intervention?

8. Identify and describe the two components of self-efficacy as it relates to the TTM.

9. When using the TTM, why is it best for health educators to use stage-matched interventions?

10. Find two research-based behavioral change intervention programs which utilized the TTM. Briefly describe the goals, methods, and outcomes of each intervention.

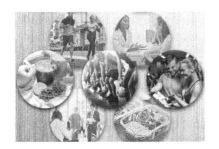

CHAPTER 7
Social Cognitive Theory

Part III of this book emphasizes interpersonal models of health behavior: Social Cognitive Theory and Social Networks/Social Support. Health behaviors are not merely based on individual factors, but a product of multiple influences or interpersonal factors. The interpersonal level focuses primarily on health behaviors which are influenced by our relationships with others and others' attitudes and behaviors. Interpersonal influences include the people within our social circle, such as family, friends, acquaintances, neighbors, teachers, coaches, and coworkers. This chapter details Social Cognitive Theory (SCT), which postulates that individuals and their environments interact with and influence each other (reciprocal determinism), resulting in individual and social change. The chapter provides information on the history and origin of SCT, a description of the constructs which comprise SCT, and an example of the application of SCT to a health promotion intervention program.

History of Social Cognitive Theory (SCT)

Most theories of behavior utilized in health promotion are concerned largely with initiating a behavioral change, and less with maintaining behavior. However, maintenance of health behavior change, and not merely the initiation of change, is the ultimate goal in health promotion. Therefore, it is important to consider behavior from a self-regulation perspective. People use a wide range of methods to self-regulate, including stimulus control and reinforcement approaches. Self-regulation provides an excellent perspective for understanding the relationships among the operant, cognitive, and social perspectives of motivation and behavior (Simons-Morton, McLeroy, & Wendel, 2012). It is the goal of Social Cognitive Theory to explain how people regulate or maintain their behavior. **Social Cognitive Theory**, used in health promotion, psychology, education, and communication, posits that portions of an individual's knowledge attainment can be directly related to the individual's observation of others relative to the context of social interactions, experiences, and outside environmental influences. One of the many features of SCT is that it offers a number of constructs, including self-efficacy and observational learning, which have been used extensively in health education/promotion, as well as in a number of other theories and models (Glanz, Rimer, & Viswanath, 2008). Selected constructs of SCT have been applied, rather than the complete theory.

SCT was built on previous theorization and research by Miller and Dollard (1941) and Rotter (1954). Social cognitive theory was first known as *social learning theory*, as it was based on principles of learning within the human social context (Bandura, 1977). It was renamed Social Cognitive Theory when concepts from cognitive psychology were integrated to accommodate the growing understanding of human information processing capacities that influence learning from experience, observation, and symbolic communication (Bandura, 1986). With further development, SCT embraced concepts from sociology and political science to improve its understanding of the adaptive capacities of groups and societies (Bandura, 1997). SCT also integrated and developed concepts from humanistic psychology by analyzing the processes that underlie self-determination, altruism (selflessness), and moral behavior (Bandura, 1999).

The development of the earliest applications of SCT followed the rejection of the prevailing theories and concepts being applied to psychotherapy, particularly the idea that individual differences in behavior resulted from personality traits. In the 1960s and 1970s, researchers began to apply behavioral and social learning concepts to the development of more effective cognitive/behavioral programs to assist people in changing or managing unwanted behaviors (Bandura, 1969; Meichenbaum, 1977). Bandura's first comprehensive textbook, *Principles of Behavior Modification*, provided a detailed analysis of a large body of evidence showing that human behavior could be modified and personally regulated based on knowledge derived from empirical studies of how people learn from and adapt to their environment (Bandura, 1969; Glanz et al., 2008). Behavior is the product of a person's learning history, perceptions of the present environment, and intellectual and physical capacities. Consequently, behavior can be changed through new learning experiences, changes in social norms and perceptions of the present environment, and the development of capacities through health promotion and behavioral change interventions.

Constructs of Social Cognitive Theory

SCT seeks to explain how our experiences, environments, and behaviors affect how we learn. Its purpose is to understand and predict individual and group behavior, as well as to identify methods whereby behavior can be modified or changed. SCT is frequently used in interventions aimed at personality development, behavioral pathology, and health promotion. SCT is based on understanding an individual's reality construct. According to SCT, learners acquire knowledge as their environment converges with personal characteristics and personal experience. New experiences are evaluated via the past; and prior experiences help to subsequently guide and inform the learner as to how the present should be investigated. The nine key concepts that comprise SCT include: (1) reciprocal determinism, (2) outcome expectations, (3) self-efficacy, (4) collective efficacy, (5) observational learning, (6) incentive motivation, (7) facilitation, (8) self-regulation, and (9) moral disengagement. Table 7.1 provides definitions of the concepts which comprise SCT.

Reciprocal Determinism

The central concept of SCT is **reciprocal determinism**, also referred to as *triadic reciprocity* (see Figure 7.1). It is defined as the dynamic interaction of the person, the behavior, and the environment in which the behavior is performed, thus facilitating self-regulation of behavior. In other words, human behavior is the product of the interplay of personal, behavioral, and environmental influences. This theory recognizes how environments

Table 7.1.   Constructs of Social Cognitive Theory.

Reciprocal Determinism	The dynamic interaction of the person, the behavior, and the environment in which the behavior is performed
Outcome Expectations	Beliefs about the likelihood and value of the consequences of behavioral choices
Self-Efficacy	The person's confidence in ability to perform behaviors that bring desired outcomes
Collective Efficacy	Beliefs about the ability of a group to perform concerted actions that bring desired outcomes
Observational Learning	Behavioral acquisition that occurs by watching the actions and outcomes of others' behavior
Incentive Motivation	The use of rewards and punishments to modify behavior
Facilitation	Providing tools, knowledge, skills, resources, or environmental changes to perform a given behavior or make new behaviors easier to perform
Self-Regulation	Personal regulation of goal-directed behavior or performance
Moral Disengagement	Strategies or tactics used by people to deal with emotional stimuli

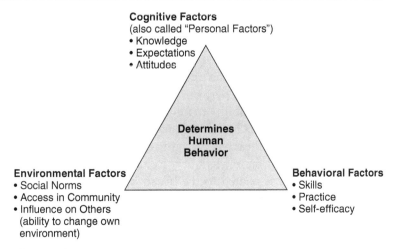

Figure 7.1. Reciprocal Determinism.

© Kendall Hunt Publishing Company.

shape behavior, but also focuses on people's potential to alter and influence environments to suit selective purposes. **Cognitive Factors** refer to the individual, with a unique personality, set of experiences, knowledge, and learned behaviors. **Environmental Factors** represent the external physical and social influences to outside stimuli and potential reinforcements. **Behavioral Factors** include responses to stimuli to achieve immediate and long-term goals. Each person responds to the environment differently, based on past experiences and personal factors. The environment influences behavior by providing context, opportunity, and feedback, which are processed and acted upon uniquely by each individual. While the environment affects health behavior, behavior also has an impact on the environment, providing unique feedback to the individual (Simons-Morton et al., 2012). Planned promotion of public health can be viewed as reciprocal determinism, because societies seek to control the environmental and social factors that influence different health behaviors and health outcomes. Figure 7.1 illustrates the three factors which comprise reciprocal determinism: (1) behavioral factors, (2) cognitive factors, and (3) environmental factors.

Example: Promotion of public health by changing environmental factors that influence health and health behavior, such as regulation of tobacco use in restaurants or minority access to health care services.

Outcome Expectations

Outcome expectations are beliefs about the likelihood and value of the consequences of behavioral choices. In other words, they comprise the anticipated consequences of a behavior. Thus they correspond to the concept of social norms in the Theory of Reasoned Action (TRA) and Theory of Planned Behavior (TPB) (see Chapter 5), which are defined as expectations about how different people will evaluate behavior and our willingness to be guided by their evaluation (Glanz et al., 2008). SCT posits that we develop impressions about the likelihood of various responses to behaviors we are considering. Accordingly, we anticipate the consequences of our actions in advance of actually engaging in the behavior, and sometimes in advance of encountering situations in which the behavior would be possible or relevant. There are specific types of generalized outcome expectations that seem to be particularly important in self-regulation. The expectation that the result of an anticipated behavior will be favorable and likely is a powerful motivator of behavior (Simons-Morton et al., 2012). Outcome expectations are typically learned in four ways: (1) performance attainment, (2) vicarious experience, (3) social persuasion, and (4) physiological arousal. **Performance attainment** deals with previous experiences in similar situations. **Vicarious experience** involves observing others in similar situations. **Social persuasion** includes hearing about situations from other people. **Physiological arousal** deals with emotional or physical responses to behaviors.

Example: Changing expectations about the pleasure associated with condom use; preventing motor vehicle accidents by not texting while driving.

Self-Efficacy

Self-efficacy (Bandura, 1997) is the concept for which SCT is most widely known, and it has been integrated into a number of other models and theories (see Chapter 4 and Chapter 6). **Self-efficacy** is defined as a person's confidence in performing a particular behavior and in overcoming barriers to that behavior. In other words, our perception about our own personal ability to perform behaviors that bring about desired outcomes. In SCT, self-efficacy refers to our confidence in our ability to undertake a specific action successfully. Self-efficacy may be influenced by our capabilities and other individual factors, as well as by environmental enablers and barriers (Simons-Morton et al., 2012). Self-efficacy is thought to be enhanced by successful experience, and undermined by failure or frustration. A common method for enhancing self-efficacy is to provide instruction and practice to mastery. Self-efficacy is related to the broad concepts of self-concept, self-esteem, and self-image. Self-efficacy is considered an essential aspect of intent, which is an important characteristic of self-directed health behavior.

SCT identifies four major ways in which self-efficacy can be developed (Bandura, 2004): (1) *mastery experience*, or enabling the person to succeed in attainable but increasingly challenging performances of desired behaviors; (2) *social modeling*, or showing the person that others similar to themselves are able to succeed in the desired behaviors; (3) *improving physical and emotional states*, or making sure the person is well-rested and physically or mentally prepared before attempting new behaviors; and (4) *verbal persuasion*, or spoken encouragement and reinforcement from others to boost confidence enough to induce the desired behaviors.

Example: Improving a person's beliefs and practice about being able to consistently use condoms when participating in sexual activity with a partner; educating pregnant women on how to properly breastfeed their baby.

Collective Efficacy

Collective efficacy refers to the beliefs about the ability of a group to perform concerted actions that bring desired outcomes. Since a number of the things that people seek are achievable only by working together with others in the community, Bandura has extended the concept of self-efficacy to collective efficacy. The quality of health as a nation is a social matter, and not just a personal one. It requires changing the practices of social systems that impair health, rather than just changing the habits of individuals. People's beliefs in their collective efficacy to accomplish social change by group action play a key role in the policy and public health approach to health promotion. Given that health is heavily influenced by behavioral, environmental, and economic factors, health promotion requires emphasis on the development and enlistment of collective efficacy for socially oriented initiatives (Bandura, 1997; Fernández-Ballesteros, Díez Nicolás, Caprara, Barbaranelli, & Bandura, 2002).

Example: Organization of parental groups to establish designated drivers to reduce underage drinking and driving on prom night; organization of local groups to promote research and awareness for a particular health cause, such as Race for the Cure for breast cancer; changes in social policies for gun reform in America.

Observational Learning

Observational learning is a behavioral acquisition that occurs by watching the actions of other people and the outcomes of their behavior. For example, children observe their parents when they eat, smoke, drink, and use or do not use seat belts, and they see the various rewards or penalties parents receive for these types of behaviors. According to Bandura, there are four processes which govern observational learning (Bandura, 1986; 2002): (1) attention, (2) retention, (3) production, and (4) motivation. These factors play different roles in different situations. For example, relative to *attention*, access to family, friends, and the media determines what behaviors a person is able to observe, while the value of the outcomes expected from the modeled behavior determines what people choose to pay attention to closely. Cognitive *retention* of a health behavior depends largely on intellectual capacities and other individual factors. *Production*, or the performance of a modeled behavior, depends largely on physical and communication skills as well as self-efficacy for performing, or learning to perform, the observed health behavior. *Motivation* is determined by outcome expectations about the benefits and barriers of the observed behavior (Glanz et al., 2008).

The term **modeling** also describes how people behave so that others will follow their example. Parents can model self-restraint with respect to anger, food, alcohol, and tobacco use. Parents can also model safety behaviors, such as seat belt use and driving the legal speed limit, so that their children will learn to behave in these ways. Modeling is not only an important concept for understanding the social environment and the influence of significant others on behavior, but also a useful method for changing behavior. For example, infant car seat use increases when hospital staff require that infants ride in a car safety seat when released from the hospital, especially when car safety seats can be purchased at the hospital (Brink & Simons-Morton, 1989); and mothers are more likely to place infants to sleep on their backs when they observe hospital staff placing infants on their backs (Brenner et al., 2003). In addition, a number of studies have shown that models are imitated most frequently when observers perceive the models to be similar in some fashion to themselves (Brody & Stoneman, 1981; Schunk, 1987). This makes peer-modeling a well-recognized method for influencing behavior, particularly among children and adolescents.

Example: Entertainment education featuring healthy adolescents who do not drink or smoke; peer education programs aimed at responsible sexual behavior and condom use.

Incentive Motivation

Incentive motivation consists of responses to a person's behavior that increase or decrease the likelihood of reoccurrence, such as the use of rewards and/or punishments to modify behavior (Glanz et al., 2008). Rewards may be extrinsic or intrinsic. **Extrinsic rewards** are regarded as the occurrence of an event that is known to have a predictable reinforcement value. Extrinsic motivation refers to the performance of an activity in order to attain an outcome. Common extrinsic motivators are money, threat of punishment, grades, awards, and encouragement from others. **Intrinsic rewards** are characterized as a person's own experience/perception that an activity had some value. Intrinsic motivation refers to motivation that is driven by an interest or enjoyment in the task itself, rather than reliance on any external influences. Intrinsically motivated people attribute their results to factors under their own control, which is also known as autonomy, and believe they have the skills that will allow them to be effective in reaching their desired goals.

Example: Examples of extrinsic rewards include increasing the taxes on tobacco products, fitting into a smaller size due to consistent physical activity, or having more money as a result of maintaining health. Examples of intrinsic rewards include feeling better about oneself for eating healthfully or enjoying being outdoors when exercising.

Facilitation

Facilitation involves providing tools, knowledge, skills, resources, or environmental changes to perform a given behavior or make new behaviors easier to perform. Motivation seeks to manipulate behavior through external control, whereas facilitation is empowering. SCT joins a number of other theories and models of health behavior in stressing the importance of recognizing barriers to behavior change and identifying ways in which those barriers can be removed or overcome.

Example: Building sidewalks to promote and increase physical activity; education about condom use for HIV protection and distribution of condoms at no cost, making condoms readily available to those with the greatest risk for STIs.

Self-Regulation

Self-regulation is defined as the personal regulation of goal-directed behavior or performance. SCT emphasizes the capacity for people to endure short-term negative outcomes in anticipation of important long-term positive outcomes (Karoly, 1993). This is achieved through self-regulation. According to SCT, self-control does not merely depend on "willpower" but instead on concrete skills for managing oneself. One of the goals of health promotion is to bring the performance of health behavior under control of the individual. Bandura (1997), identified six ways in which self-regulation is achieved: (1) *self-monitoring*, or systematic observation of one's own behavior; (2) *goal-setting*, or the identification of short-term and long-term changes; (3) *feedback*, or information about the quality of performance and how it may be improved; (4) *self-reward*, or one's provision of tangible or intangible rewards for oneself; (5) *self-instruction*, or talking to oneself or preparing before and during the performance of a complex behavior; and (6) *social support*, as when one has other people to encourage one's efforts to exert self-control.

Example: Computerized training programs for patients with diabetes; counseling services for smoking cessation or other substance abuse issues; rewarding oneself at the end of the week for adhering to a planned diet and exercise regime.

Moral Disengagement

Moral disengagement includes strategies or tactics used by a person to deal with emotional stimuli. SCT describes how people can learn moral standards for self-regulation that can lead them to avoid violence and cruelty toward others. Moral disengagement involves ways of thinking about harmful behaviors and the people who are harmed that make infliction of suffering acceptable by disengaging self-regulatory moral standards. People can violate standards of self-regulation through what Bandura (1999) labels as mechanisms of moral disengagement. These include: *euphemistic labeling*, which sanitizes acts of violence by using words that make them less offensive; *dehumanization and attribution of blame* to victims, perceiving them as racially or ethnically different and at fault for the punishment they receive; *diffusion and displacement of responsibility* by attributing decisions to a group or to authority figures; and *perceived moral justification* for harmful behaviors by construing them as beneficial and/or necessary. Psychological defenses, cognitive techniques, stress management, advocating for health issues, or other methods for solving problems effectively are all examples of tactics to ameliorate moral disengagement.

Example: Dehumanization and diffusion of responsibility that may harm public health, such as poverty, starvation, marketing of tobacco products, and access to health care services.

Application of Social Cognitive Theory

SCT is a comprehensive framework based upon a large pool of empirical evidence which provides insight into factors that influence human behavior and learning. For health education, SCT serves to meet challenges that arise when designing and implementing health promotion programs or interventions. As previously noted, some health interventions apply select constructs of SCT rather than the complete theory. SCT has been applied to a broad range of approaches to modify diverse health behaviors. Following is an example of how SCT has been applied to a smoking-cessation telephone counseling intervention.

Beginning in June of 2000, the American Cancer Society (ACS) applied the SCT construct of self-regulation to a telephone smoking-cessation counseling service in the state of Texas. The goal of the service was to help smokers quit tobacco by using self-regulation as a guide. Subsequently, the counseling service was adopted by other states and organizations. The program was administered by paraprofessional counselors, such as smoking-cessation specialists, who had received approximately 140 hours of training. The counselors were guided by computer screens which incorporated scripts based on decision trees in the counseling protocol. Ultimately, this service provided assistance to over 250,000 smokers. In a randomized clinical trial, the ACS telephone counseling service was shown to almost double a smoker's likelihood of staying tobacco-free for one year, as compared to smokers who utilized self-help booklets from the mall (McAlister et al., 2004). The decision trees in the ACS protocol included elements addressing the six self-regulatory processes in SCT: (1) self-monitoring, (2) goal setting, (3) feedback, (4) self-reward, (5) self-instruction, and (6) social support. Table 7.2 provides an example of the application of SCT to a smoking-cessation program.

Self-Monitoring

Self-monitoring is the effective systematic observation of one's own behavior, including observing and recording both the behavior itself and the context and cues or events that accompany the behavior. In the ACS telephone counseling service, this was done by having clients keep simple records of their smoking and the context and cues that were present when they smoked. This enabled clients to identify any triggers that caused them to smoke and led to the development of effective coping skills which would be necessary during the cessation process.

Goal Setting

Goal setting is a planned behavior in which intentions are formulated in terms of both short-term and long-term goals in order to bring people closer to the changes they desire (Glanz et al., 2008). Gradual steps are

Table 7.2. Social Cognitive Theory (SCT): Application to a Smoking-Cessation Program.

Concept	Intervention
Self-Monitoring	Recording date and time of smoking and the context and cues present when smoking
Goal Setting	Setting short-term goals (1 day) and longer-term goals (1 week) for quitting cigarette smoking
Feedback	Internal and external information gathered regarding attempts at quitting smoking
Self-Reward	Short-term and longer-term rewards of saving money by not purchasing cigarettes
Self-Instruction	Instructing oneself on stress management techniques, such as deep breathing exercises to reduce cravings for tobacco
Social Support	Enlisting social support (family, friends, coworkers) to increase self-efficacy, feedback, and cues to action

needed in order to build self-efficacy. Short-term goals may be one day, one week, or one month in duration. Long-term goals are typically measured in longer durations, such as six months, one year, or three to five years. In the ACS telephone counseling program, the initial objective for a smoker trying to quit was a single day of not smoking. When that was achieved, the next goal would be to not smoke for three days. Goals were created depending on the client's progress.

Feedback

Feedback consists of information regarding the quantity and quality of the behavior being learned, as provided by others and from one's own observations. In the ACS telephone counseling program, this typically occurred when stress would trigger a client to relapse. Clients were instructed to utilize positive relaxation techniques in anticipation of future stressors that might cause them to revert back to smoking. To order to maintain self-efficacy, both internal and external feedback on an unsuccessful performance should be framed positively rather than be treated as a failure. Clients in the program were encouraged to learn and benefit from the experience in their next effort to quit.

Self-Reward

In the early stages of the self-management process, the short-term rewards people give to themselves may be more effective than the long-term rewards they gain in the future. In the ACS telephone counseling program, clients were encouraged to set aside part of their savings from not purchasing cigarettes for weekly pleasures, while saving the rest for a more expensive gratification at the end of the month. Clients were encouraged to actively reward themselves for their progress. The most immediate form of self-reward is the feeling of satisfaction from making progress.

Self-Instruction

Self-instruction involves effectively speaking to oneself about each subtask in a series of tasks. In the ACS telephone counseling program, clients were guided through multiple rehearsals of a combination of diaphragmatic breathing and self-instruction to help them cope with stress and reduce tobacco cravings. Self-instructions are also formulated and rehearsed for other situations that may cause relapse, such as social occasions where alcohol is offered and people are smoking tobacco.

Social Support

Social Support serves multiple functions in the behavior change process. These include verbal persuasion to increase self-efficacy, provision of feedback, and direct cues to action. The ACS telephone counseling protocol required clients to identify sources of social support and to actively seek their support during the counseling process. The ACS counselors also served as short-term social support, and their training focused on ways to increase clients' self-efficacy through the provision of positive feedback.

Summary

This chapter details Social Cognitive Theory (SCT), one of the preeminent theoretical perspectives for health promotion research and practice. SCT postulates that individuals and their environments interact with and influence each other (reciprocal determinism), resulting in individual and social change. SCT seeks to provide a comprehensive understanding of both why and how people change personal health behaviors, as well as the social and physical environments that influence them. The theory includes nine key concepts: (1) reciprocal determinism, (2) outcome expectations, (3) self-efficacy, (4) collective efficacy, (5) observational learning, (6) incentive motivation, (7) facilitation, (8) self-regulation, and (9) moral disengagement. SCT fits well with other theories and it is not uncommon in practice for SCT to be paired with other theories and/or models in different programs. This chapter provided content on the history of SCT, a description and example of each of the constructs, and an example of the application of SCT to a health promotion intervention program.

References

Bandura, A. (1969). *Principles of behavior modification*. New York: Holt, Rinehart, & Winston.

Bandura, A. (1977). *Social learning theory*. Englewood Cliffs, NJ: Prentice-Hall.

Bandura, A. (1986). *Social foundations of thought and action: A social cognitive theory*. Englewood Cliffs, NJ: Prentice-Hall.

Bandura, A. (1997). *Self-efficacy: The exercise of control*. New York: Freeman.

Bandura, A. (1999). Moral disengagement in the perpetration of inhumanities. *Personality & Social Psychology Review, 3*, 193–209.

Bandura, A. (2002). Social cognitive theory of mass communications. In J. Bryant & D. Zillman (Eds.), *Media effects: Advances in theory and research* (2nd ed.). Hillsdale, NJ: Erlbaum.

Bandura, A. (2004). Health promotion by social cognitive means. *Health Education & Behavior, 31*, 143–164.

Brenner, R. A., Simons-Morton, B. G., Bhaskar, B., Revenis, M., Das, A., & Clemens, J. (2003). Infant-parent bed sharing in an inner-city population. *Archives of Pediatrics & Adolescent Medicine, 157*, 33–39.

Brink, S. G., & Simons-Morton, B. G. (1989). Evaluation of a hospital-based car safety seat education and loan program for low-income mothers: The Car Seat Connection. *Health Education Quarterly, 16*, 45–56.

Brody, G. H., & Stoneman, Z. (1981). Selective imitation of same-sex, older and younger peer models. *Child Development, 52*, 717–720.

Fernández-Ballesteros, R., Díez Nicolás, J., Caprara, G. V., Barbaranelli, C., & Bandura, A. (2002). Self-efficacy and collective efficacy: Structural relationships. *Applied Psychology: An International Review. 51*, 107–121.

Glanz, K., Rimer, B. K., & Viswanath, K. (2008). *Health behavior and health education: Theory, research, and practice* (4th ed.). San Francisco: John Wiley.

Karoly, P. (1993). Mechanisms of self-regulation. *Annual Review of Psychology, 44*, 23–52.

McAlister, A. L., Rabius, V., Geiger, A., Glynn, T. J., Huang, P., & Todd, R. (2004). Telephone assistance for smoking cessation: One year cost effectiveness estimations. *Tobacco Control, 13*, 85–86.

Meichenbaum, D. (1977). *Cognitive-behavior modification: An integrative approach*. New York: Plenum.

Miller, N. E., & Dollard, J. (1941). *Social learning and imitation*. New Haven: Yale University Press.

Rotter, J. B. (1954). *Social learning and clinical psychology*. Englewood Cliffs, NJ: Prentice-Hall.

Schunk, D. H. (1987). Peer models and children's behavioral changes. *Review of Educational Research, 57*, 149–174.

Simons-Morton, B., McLeroy, K., & Wendel, M. (2012). *Behavior theory in health promotion practice and research*. Burlington, MA: Jones & Bartlett Learning.

Chapter 7—Review Questions

1. Describe the differences between intrapersonal models and interpersonal models.

2. Briefly describe how Social Cognitive Theory (SCT) evolved into the theory it is today.

3. Define reciprocal determinism. Explain how person, behavior, and environment interact according to this SCT construct.

4. What are outcome expectations and how are they learned?

5. Compare and contrast self-efficacy and collective efficacy. Provide an example for each.

6. Explain the processes of observational learning and provide an example of each.

7. What are the two types of rewards provided by incentive motivation? Provide an example for each.

8. Identify and define the six regulatory processes in SCT.

9. Identify and define the six ways in which self-regulation is achieved. Provide an example for each.

10. What are the four mechanisms of moral disengagement identified by Bandura?

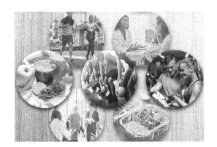

CHAPTER 8
Social Networks and Social Support

The correlation between social relationships and health has become a focal point in the practice of health education. As previously stated in this text, health behavior and health decision-making are often influenced by family, friends, and coworkers. It is necessary for health educators to understand the impact of social networks and social support on an individual's overall health status. While there is no one theory which thoroughly summarizes the implications of social relationships for health status, various theories used in research have provided empirical support for this link. This chapter will explore the components of social networks and social support, provide evidence on how behavior is produced by social influences, and present an applied example related to the obesity epidemic.

History

In the 1950s, British anthropologists found it difficult to understand the behavior of individuals and groups based on traditional categories of kin groups, tribes, and villages (Berkman, Glass, Brissette, & Seeman, 2000). Barnes (1954) developed the concept of social networks, which described patterns of social relationships across traditional kinship, residential, and class groups, through his work in a Norwegian village. Early research on social networks was qualitative and exploratory in nature. The development of social network theories and models provided a way to examine the properties of relationships among individuals, with no expectation that these relationships were present only in extended families or work groups.

Analysis of social networks "focuses on the characteristic patterns of ties between actors in a social system rather than on characteristics of the individual actors themselves and uses these descriptions to study how these social structures constrain network members' behavior" (Hall & Wellman, 1985). Additionally, network analysis examines the composition of the network and the resources which are provided by networks. Social network theories assume that the structure of the social network is responsible for determining individual behavior and attitudes by controlling the availability of resources which, in turn, influence behavior. In other words, the availability or lack of availability of resources for an individual provides both behavioral and affective responses. Furthermore, Bott (1957) indicated that social networks may not conform to traditional notions of community as defined by geographic location or family ties through her examination of families in London. Examining the links between social network members can help determine which characteristics comprise the community (i.e., geographic location, family ties, friendship, work groups, etc.) (Berkman et al., 2000).

Social Networks

Social network refers to the extent to which an individual is connected with others (Simons-Morton, McLeroy, & Wendel, 2012). A network provides patterns of advice, communication, and support that exist between members of a social structure (Valente, 1995; Scott, 2000). Social networks are composed of structural characteristics and relational characteristics. Table 8.1 provides definitions for each structural and relational characteristic.

Table 8.1.   Social Network Characteristics.

Structural Characteristics	Definition
Formality	Degree to which social relationships are present in the framework of organizational or institutional roles
Density	Degree to which network members are acquainted and intermingle with each other
Homogeneity	Degree to which network members are demographically equivalent
Geographic Dispersion	Degree to which network members reside close to the focal individual
Relational Characteristics	**Definition**
Reciprocity	Degree to which resources and support are given as well as received in a relationship
Intensity/Strength	Degree to which relationships offer affective support
Complexity	Degree to which social relationships provide multiple roles
Directionality	Degree to which network members share equal parts of power and influence

Structural characteristics include: (1) formality, (2) density, (3) homogeneity, and (4) geographic dispersion which provides information regarding the network as a whole. The characteristic of **formality** is the extent to which social relationships exist in the context of organizational or institutional roles (Heaney & Israel, 2008). The extent to which social network members know each other and have multiple interactions refers to the **density** of a social network. When measuring the demographics of social networks, **homogeneity** is the extent to which the members of the social network are demographically similar. Relative to geographic location and living situation, the extent to which network members live close to the focal individual incorporates the characteristic of **geographic dispersion**.

Relational characteristics include: (1) reciprocity, (2) intensity/strength, (3) complexity, and (4) directionality which provides information regarding the relationships between the focal individual and others in the social network. Specifically, **reciprocity** is the extent to which support is offered and received among social network members. The **intensity/strength** of a social network incorporates the extent to which social network members offer affective support. When studying the **complexity** of social networks, researchers look at the extent to which social network members serve many functions within the network. The characteristic of **directionality** refers to the extent to which network members share equal amounts of power and influence during their social interactions.

Social networks encompass every person with whom an individual has contact, interacts, or exchanges information. Typically, social networks include family, close friends, coworkers, teachers, coaches, and acquaintances. The size of a social network varies from person to person; some social networks can be more extensive than others. As an individual's life situation changes, their social network also evolves (Bidart & Lavenu, 2005). For example, going away to college, starting a new job, or moving across the country are life events which can expand or reduce a social network. Social networks can be sustained through various mediums such as the Internet, telephone, or travel. Social networks provide individuals with important social functions, such as social support, social capital, and social influence.

Research suggests there is an important relationship between the health status of individuals and their social relationships or social network (House, 1987). According to Cassel (1976), the positive impact social relationships have on health is not disease specific. Even though there have been inconsistencies in research findings regarding the link between social networks/social support and specific diseases, affective support provided during recovery from serious illness has been consistently documented (Spiegle & Diamond, 2001; Wang, Mittleman, & Orth-Gomer, 2005). In other words, individuals suffering from disease, whether it is chronic or infectious, will benefit from the support they receive from their social network members. More specifically, epidemiological studies indicate there is a correlation between a lack of social network ties and all causes of mortality (Berkman & Glass, 2000). Recently, studies have found that the affective support provided by intimate ties increases the survival rate of individuals with severe cardiovascular disease (Berkman et al., 2000). Additionally, individuals who have at least one strong intimate social relationship tend to be in good health (Michael, Colditz, Coakley, & Kawanchi, 1999). In a five-year study with elderly Black women, researchers found that severe social isolation was correlated with a threefold increase in the mortality rate among the study participants (La Veist, Sellers, Brown, & Nickerson, 1997).

Social Support

Social support is a concept which incorporates receiving help from others during a difficult life event. Cobb (1976) defined **social support** as "the individual belief that one is cared for and loved, esteemed and valued, and belongs to a network of communication and mutual obligations." The provision of social support is a key component in social relationships (Burg & Seeman, 1994). Social support is distinguishable from all other functions of social relationships because it is intended to be helpful, it is consciously provided, and it manifests from caring, trust, and respect. Since social support is given consciously, it is different from social influence, which manifests from observation of others' behavior (Bandura, 1986) and from receiver-initiated social comparison (Wood, 1996).

House (1981) identified four types of social support that compose the functional capacity of relationships: (1) emotional support, (2) instrumental support, (3) informational support, and (4) appraisal support. **Emotional support** is the provision of empathy, love, trust, and concern. Emotional support is the most commonly recognized form of social support. It is typically provided by family and close friends. **Instrumental support** is the provision of concrete aid or services that directly impact the individual in need. Financial assistance is considered instrumental support. **Informational support** is the provision of advice, information, or suggestions that would be useful to the individual in need. A clinic that provides informational pamphlets to patients provides them with informational support. **Appraisal support** is the provision of information in the form of feedback. Appraisal support is evaluative in nature and is usually given by family, close friends, teachers, and coaches. Even though there are definitive differences between the four types of social support, if a relationship provides one type of social support, it will usually provide other types as well. While social support provides physical and mental support to individuals, social networks provide a basis for intimacy and attachment. Intimacy and attachment are not only experienced between family and friends, but can also be experienced through extended social relationships. For example, when there is a strong relationship with community, an individual may feel intimacy and attachment to neighbors and/or other community organizations.

Figure 8.1 illustrates the interplay between social support and social networks. As shown, environmental and personal factors contribute to the characteristics (structural and relational) that comprise a personal social

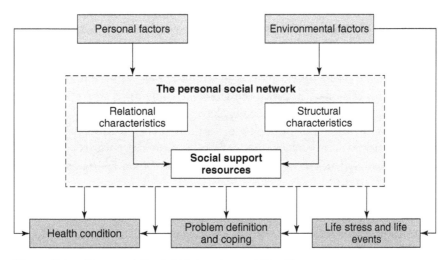

Figure 8.1. Personal Social Networks and Health.

network. This particular model demonstrates that social support is a result of the social network characteristics working together. There is a clear distinction between the characteristics of the social network and the social support an individual receives. When a person perceives a stressful event, the social network and social support can help in addressing the stressful event by defining the problem and establishing an adequate coping technique or treatment for the problem. An individuals social network and social support can also help by providing emotional, informational, or instrumental support to assist in treating a health condition.

Social Capital

Social capital refers to the connectedness within and among social networks. It is concerned with the context and depth of social relationships. Social capital theory is prominent in the practice of health education (Kreuter & Lezin, 2002). **Social Capital Theory** posits that social networks have value (Putnam, 2000). This concept is based upon the observed benefits of being part of a social system (Simons-Morton et al., 2012). There are three key components of social capital that make it valuable: trust, reciprocity, and cooperation. The presence and absence of social capital has been linked to depression, child welfare, violent behavior, mortality, and overall health status (Kawachi, Kennedy, & Glass, 1999; Putnam, 2000). Morbidity from chronic diseases such as diabetes and obesity decreases within communities when social capital increases (Holtgrave & Crosby, 2006). Additionally, infectious diseases and illnesses, such as sexually transmitted infections (STIs), have been shown to decrease within a community when the amount of social capital increases (Holtgrave & Crosby, 2003).

Social Influence

Social influence is the byproduct of information sharing among network members that leads to common social norms. "In this context, **information** refers to input from all available sources about a particular thought or behavior" (Simons-Morton et al., 2012). The social norms that result from social influence are the knowledge, attitudes, behaviors, and values a social network holds. It is through social norms that social influence affects health behaviors. Under conditions of uncertainty, "people obtain normative guidance by comparing their attitudes with those of a reference group of similar others. Attitudes are conformed and reinforced when they are shared with the comparison group but altered when they are discrepant" (Marsden & Friedkin, 1994). Social norms regarding health behaviors may be powerful sources of social influence which directly influence the behavior of network members. For example, cigarette smoking among peers is one of the best predictors of smoking initiation among adolescents (Landrine, Richardson, Klondoff, & Flay, 1994).

Social norms are attitudes, behaviors, and values which are perceived to be true and acceptable within a social network. Social norms can vary between social networks. Social norms dictate behavior through the concept of conformity. Research indicates that most individuals will go along with the group majority rather than against the majority, even if they do not agree with the majority (Asch, 1955; Forgas & Williams, 2001). Individuals who are highly independent tend to be rejected or ridiculed by social groups, which dissuades them from being assertive (Levine, 1989). Therefore, social norms influence behavior by creating standards and expectations that individuals may choose to accept or reject.

There are two types of social influence: normative and informational (Aronson, Wilson, & Akert, 1999). **Normative influence** is concerned with being accepted or approved by others. Individuals who exert normative influence are constantly trying to please others in order to receive appreciation or praise from network members. **Informational influence** is concerned with always being correct. Individuals who exert informational influence are constantly correcting others because they believe they have all the right answers. Group membership in families, friend cliques, organizations, and professions all provide individuals with a set of social norms. Group memberships enforce normative behavior among group members by means of rewards and punishments. Figure 8.2 provides an example of a social network in which a professor has the potential to positively influence students.

Social Network and Social Support Interventions

Several types of interventions focus on social networks and social support; this text will focus on the four main types: (1) enhancing existing network support, (2) developing new social network ties, (3) enhancing existing network support by using natural helpers and community health workers, and (4) enhancing network support

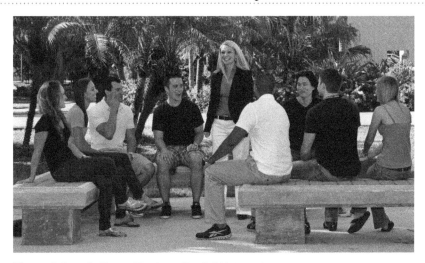

Figure 8.2. College Student Social Network.

through community capacity building and problem solving. Table 8.2 depicts the four categories of interventions and provides descriptions of possible intervention strategies.

Interventions aimed at enhancing existing network support attempt to change the attitudes and behaviors of the support providers, the support receivers, or both. To effectively enhance existing social ties, health educators must identify social network members who are willing to commit to providing support and resources when necessary. Additionally, health educators must identify which attitudes and behaviors must change to provide the support recipient with the greatest increase in perceived social support.

Interventions which focus on developing new social network ties are most effective when an individual's social network is small, overburdened, or cannot provide effective support (Heaney & Israel, 2008). The use of "mentors" or "advisers" offers program participants the opportunity to receive support from an individual who has already experienced what the participant is currently experiencing. Self-help groups are effective at creating new social ties because individuals in these groups tend to be facing the same life stressors and can offer encouragement and support to one another.

Natural helpers are individuals within a social network who provide support, encouragement, and advice to others. Natural-helper interventions must first identify which individuals fill the helping role within a social

Table 8.2. Social Network and Social Support Interventions and Strategies

Intervention Type	Intervention Strategies
Enhancing existing network support	• Activities to build skills for support mobilization, provision, and receipt • Enhance the quality of social ties
Developing new social network ties	• Use "mentors" or "advisers" to create new support ties • Use a buddy system to link individuals together to increase available support
Enhancing existing network support by using natural helpers and community health workers	• Identify and recruit natural helpers or community health workers to provide continual support
Enhancing network support through community capacity building and problem solving	• Identify overlapping networks within the community • Examine the characteristics of social network members • Facilitate continual community problem-solving

network. Once natural helpers are recruited, community health workers are able to establish a consultative relationship that will benefit the community as a whole. Typically, this type of intervention focuses on community building and community problem-solving.

Involving community members in interventions that focus on community problem-solving may increase the strength of the community's social network. Interventions which utilize community organizing techniques often enhance community problem-solving and increase the community's capacity for decision-making. When community members come together to focus on a community problem, new social network ties are forged. This type of intervention usually produces an indirect effect on social networks and social support.

Application of Social Network and Social Support

When determining the effect of social relationships on health, it is advantageous to take a broader approach and examine the entire social network rather than just focus on social support. Using a social network approach allows health educators to address the multiple functions of social relationships instead of just the one function of social support (Berkman et al., 2000; Israel, 1982). Focusing on social support means that only one relationship can be studied at a time, whereas, a social network approach can address how changes to social relationships affect other social relationships (Heaney & Israel, 2008). A social network approach also allows for examination of the quality and quantity of social support an individual gives and receives (McLeroy, Gottlieb, & Heaney, 2001).

When creating social network interventions, it is important to tailor the intervention to the needs and resources of the program participants. Having program participants identify the strengths and weaknesses of their social network optimizes the effectiveness of the intervention. Most effective social network interventions utilize an ecological framework which addresses the multiple levels of influence a social network exerts on an individual (McLeroy et al., 2001). Support-enhancing interventions that motivate an individual to participate in healthy behaviors also motivate healthy change within the individual's social network. The following is an example of how social networks, social support, and social influence have impacted the obesity epidemic.

Christakis and Fowler (2007) proposed that the obesity epidemic is socially influenced. They found that the likelihood of an individual's becoming obese increases when one of the members of the individual's social network becomes obese. Additionally, nonobese individuals have a higher risk of becoming obese when there are high numbers of obese members in their social network. Social proximity increased the likelihood of an individual's becoming obese by twofold if the individual was in constant contact with an obese person. There was also a greater affect between same-sex individuals in the social network rather than opposite-sex individuals with regard to becoming obese. These results revealed that the transference of social norms regarding weight management typically occurred between same-sex individuals. Furthermore, the likelihood of weight loss increased if one of the obese members of the social network lost weight.

Christakis and Fowler (2007) provided empirical evidence indicating that the nature of friendship also affects obesity within social networks. In order to become obese, an individual must be friends with an obese individual, not just a friend of a friend of such a person. The likelihood of obesity was greatest among reciprocal friendships, prominent among those who identified an obese person as a friend even though the friendship was not reciprocated by the obese person, and very low among obese individuals who indicated a friendship that was not reciprocated by the other person. More simply, the risk of becoming obese was greater if the individual had an obese friend or indicated an obese person as a friend, than if an obese person indicated himself or herself as a friend. Christakis and Fowler concluded that obese people increase the prevalence of obesity in their social network by either changing the acceptability of being overweight or by directly or indirectly influencing the amount of food consumed by members of the social network.

There are multiple explanations for the relationships Christakis and Fowler (2007) found, but all the explanations are influenced by social norms. Obese individuals within a social network experience the social contexts which promote obesity as a norm. Obese individuals also associate with other obese individuals who share the same social norms regarding obesity, food consumption, and exercise. Lastly, obese individuals may exert intentional or unintentional pressure on members of their social network by causing them to overeat or making obesity normative within the social network. Regardless of the explanation, Christakis and Fowler's research reiterates the influence social networks and social support have on health behavior.

Summary

Social relationships exert a large amount of influence on overall health status. Research indicates that individuals who maintain long-term social relationships have a higher quantity and quality of life. Social networks influence our health behaviors and health decision-making by providing means of social support, social capital, and social influence. Social support can be provided to an individual in need through (1) emotional, (2) instrumental, (3) informational, and (4) appraisal means. Social capital refers to the concept of connectedness between individuals in a social network. Social Capital Theory emphasizes the importance of social capital by postulating that social capital has value. The extent to which social influence manipulates health behavior relies heavily on the social norms of the network members. Interventions aimed at increasing social support can be successful at creating healthy behaviors in both individuals and social networks. When creating interventions related to social relationships and health status, health educators may choose either a social support or a social network approach to promote health among individuals and social networks. In addition, health educators can strengthen the social network of a community either by using natural helpers or by encouraging community members to get involved with community problem-solving.

References

Aronson, E., Wilson, T. D., & Akert, R. M. (1999). *Social psychology.* New York: Addison-Wesley.

Asch, S. E. (1955). Opinions and social pressure. *Scientific American, 193,* 31–35.

Bandura, A. (1986). *Social foundations of thought and action.* Englewood Cliffs, NJ: Prentice-Hall.

Barnes, J. A. (1954). Class and committees in a Norwegian island parish. *Human Relations, 7,* 39–58.

Berkman, L. F., & Glass, T. (2000). Social integration, social networks, social support, and health. In L. F. Berkman & I. Kawachi (Eds.), *Social epidemiology.* New York: Oxford University Press.

Berkman, L. F., Glass, T., Brissette, I., & Seeman, T. E. (2000). From social integration to health: Durkheim in the new millennium. *Social Science and Medicine, 51,* 843–857.

Bidart, C., & Lavenu, D. (2005). Evolutions of personal networks and life events. *Social Network, 27,* 359–376.

Bott, E. (1957). *Family and social network.* London: Tavistock Press.

Burg, M. M., & Seeman, T. E. (1994). Families and health: The negative side of social ties. *Annuals of Behavioral Medicine, 16,* 109–115.

Cassel, J. (1976). The contribution of the social environment to host resistance. *American Journal of Epidemiology, 104,* 107–123.

Christakis, N. A., & Fowler, J. H. (2007). The spread of obesity in a large social network over 32 years. *New England Journal of Medicine, 357,* 370–379.

Cobb, S. (1976). Social support as moderator of life stress. *Psychosomatic Medicine, 38,* 300–314.

Forgas, J. P., & Williams, K. D. (2001). *Social influence: Direct and indirect processes.* Philadelphia: Psychology Press.

Hall, A., & Wellman, B. (1985). Social networks and social support. In S. Cohen & S. L. Syme (Eds.), *Social support and health* (pp. 23–41). Orlando, FL: Academic Press.

Heaney, C. A., & Israel, B. A. (2008). Social networks and social support. In K. Glanz, B. K. Rimer, & K. Viswanath (Eds.), *Health behavior and health education: Theory, research, and practice* (4th ed., pp. 189–210). San Francisco: Jossey-Bass.

Holtgrave, D. R., & Crosby, R. A. (2003). Social capital, poverty, and income inequalities as predictors of gonorrhea, syphilis, chlamydia and AIDS case rates in the United States. *Sexually Transmitted Infections, 79,* 62–64.

Holtgrave, D. R., & Crosby, R. A. (2006). Is social capital a protective factor against obesity and diabetes? Findings from an exploratory study. *Annals of Epidemiology, 16,* 406–408.

House, J. S. (1981). Occupational stress and coronary heart disease: A review and theoretical integration. *Journal of Health and Social Behavior, 15,* 12–27.

House, J. S. (1987). Social support and social structure. *Sociological Forum, 2,* 135–146.

Israel, B. A. (1982). Social networks and health status: Linking theory, research, and practice. *Patient Counseling and Health Education, 4,* 65–79.

Kawachi, I., Kennedy, B., & Glass, R. (1999). Social capital and self-rated health: A contextual analysis. *American Journal of Public Health, 89,* 1187–1193.

Kreuter, M. W., & Lezin, N. A. (2002). Social capital theory: Implications for community-based health promotion. In R. J. DiClemente, R. A. Crosby, & M. C. Kegler (Eds.), *Emerging theories in health promotion practice and research.* San Francisco: Jossey-Bass/Wiley.

Landrine, H., Richardson, J. K., Klondoff, E. A., & Flay, B. (1994). Cultural diversity in the predictors of adolescent cigarette smoking: The relative influence of peers. *Journal of Behavioral Medicine, 17,* 331–336.

La Veist, T. A., Sellers, R. M., Brown, K. A., & Nickerson, K. J. (1997). Extreme social isolation, use of community-based senior support services, and mortality among African American women. *American Journal of Community Psychology, 25,* 721–732.

Levine, J. M. (1989). Reaction to opinion deviance in small groups. In P. B. Paulus (Ed.), *Psychology of group influence* (2nd ed., pp. 187–231). Hillsdale, NJ: Erlbaum.

Marsden, P. V., & Friedkin, N. E. (1994). Network studies of social influence. In S. Wasserman, & J. Galaskiewicz (Eds.), *Advances in social network analysis: Research in the social and behavioral sciences* (pp. 3–25). Thousand Oaks, CA: Sage.

McLeroy, K. R., Gottlieb, N. H., & Heaney, C. A. (2001). Social health. In M. P. O'Donnell & J. S. Harris (Eds.), *Health promotion in the workplace* (3rd ed.). Albany, NY: Delmar.

Michael, Y. L., Colditz, G. A., Coakley, E., & Kawanchi, I. (1999). Health behaviors, social networks, and healthy aging: Cross-sectional evidence from the nurses' health study. *Quality of Life Research, 8,* 711–722.

Putnam, R. D. (2000). *Bowling alone: The collapse and revival of American community*. New York: Touchstone.

Scott, J. (2000). *Social network analysis: A handbook* (2nd ed.). London: Sage.

Simons-Morton, B., McLeroy, K., & Wendel, M. (2012). *Behavior theory in health promotion practice and research*. Burlington, MA: Jones & Bartlett Learning.

Spigel, D., & Diamond, S. (2001). Psychosocial interventions in cancer group therapy techniques. In A. Baum & B. L. Andersen (Eds.), *Psychosocial interventions for cancer*. Washington, DC: American Psychological Association.

Valente, T. W. (1995). *Network models of the diffusion of innovations*. Cresskill, NH: Hampton Press.

Wang, H. X., Mittleman, M., & Orth-Gomber, K. (2005). Influence of social support on progression of coronary artery disease in women. *Social Sciences and Medicine, 60,* 599–607.

Wood, J. V. (1996). What is social comparison and how should we study it? *Personality and Social Psychology Bulletin, 22,* 520–537.

Chapter 8—Review Questions

1. Define social network. Think about your social network. What types of individuals are typically found in social networks?

2. Identify the four structural and four relational characteristics of social networks. Provide a definition for each characteristic.

3. What social functions do social networks provide for individuals? Why is it important for individuals to experience these functions?

4. What are the research findings regarding social network support and specific diseases or conditions?

5. Compare and contrast the four different types of social support. Provide an example for each type.

6. What does social capital measure? Why is social capital important to a community's social network?

7. Define social influence. What part does social influence play in an individual's health status?

8. Compare and contrast normative influence and informational influence. Provide an example scenario in which an individual would exert these types of influence.

9. Describe the four categories of social network and social support interventions. How do they differ from one another?

10. What are some similarities and differences between interventions that focus on social support versus interventions that take a social network approach?

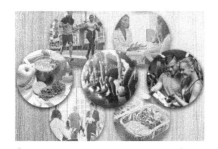

CHAPTER 9
Diffusion of Innovations

Part IV of this book emphasizes community models of health behavior: Diffusion of Innovations; Community Organization and Community Building; and Social Marketing. Major objectives of community-based interventions include community change and building capacity to address community health problems. Community-level models of health promotion focus on leadership, citizen participation, resources, skills, interpersonal networks, as well as community history, power, values, and the ability to reflect on community problems and solutions. For example, there has been a dramatic increase in health promotion programs, including smoking-cessation, physical activity, and safety programs carried out by community organizations, such as churches, health care clinics, YMCAs, and other local or state cancer and heart disease associations. The community level of the ecological perspective also works to target social conditions, such as unemployment, poverty, housing, gangs/violence, drug and alcohol use, physical inactivity, obesity, school drop out rates, adolescent pregnancy, and STIs. This chapter details the Diffusion of Innovations theory— how ideas and practices are adopted over time. The chapter provides information on the history and origin of Diffusion of Innovations, a description of the key concepts that comprise diffusion theory, and an example of the application of Diffusion of Innovations.

History of Diffusion of Innovations

The Diffusion of Innovations theory developed out of research looking backward in time at the rate of adoption of innovations and the characteristics of the innovations as well as the adopters. Some innovations spread rapidly, while the adoption of other innovations become stagnant. The history of innovations teaches us that it often takes too long for proven concepts and programs to become part of practice. For example, citrus juice was shown to be effective in preventing scurvy in 1601; however, the British navy did not introduce citrus juice into sailors' diets until nearly two centuries later in 1795 (Mosteller, 1981). Diffusion of effective programs and ideas continues to be a major challenge for public health and health promotion. Research-based interventions are often difficult to conduct in less-controlled community settings, and the research base is often not adequate to meet practitioners' needs (Oldenburg, Sallis, French, & Owen, 1999). Practitioners and policymakers want strategies and interventions that can solve major problems in their communities (Glanz, Rimer, & Viswanath, 2008). The Diffusion of Innovations theory has been used over several decades to understand the steps and processes required to achieve widespread dissemination and diffusion of public health innovations.

Much of the early research on innovations was conducted in the field of agriculture. For example, an early study by Ryan and Gross (1943) plotted the rate of adoption by Iowa farmers of a new variety of hybrid corn that had the advantage of being more resistant to pests and disease as compared to the current seeds. Over a 15-year time period, hybrid corn was adopted by the majority of Iowa farmers. Some farmers adopted the hybrid corn early, while other farmers started using the hybrid corn much later. When adoption was plotted over time, the cumulative rates of adoption created an S-shaped curve, with about 10% of farmers planting the hybrid corn in the first five years, 40% within another three years, and the remainder over the next 10 or more years. The phenomenon whereby some people adopt new practices early, others later on, and still others much later has been observed with respect to many health promotion innovations. Among the many health innovations that have been adopted according to the S-shaped curve pattern are vaccinations, fluoridated water, dental flossing, breast cancer screening, safety belt use, bicycle helmet use, and condom use.

The development of diffusion studies has emerged from multiple conceptual and research models over the last 50 years. Rogers (2003) noted in the fifth edition of his book *Diffusion of Innovations* that there were over 5,200 publications on the diffusion of diverse innovations including technology, fertility-control methods, policy innovations, consumer products, educational curricula, agricultural practices, political reforms, and health promotion programs. Rogers (2003) indicated four major research areas that account for nearly two-thirds of all diffusion publications: rural sociology, marketing and management, communication, and public health. Based on earlier approaches, three recent research areas have developed: (1) development studies, where emphasis is placed on the political, technological, or ideological context of the innovation; (2) health promotion studies, where positive health behavior is introduced and promoted as a lifestyle; and (3) evidence-based medicine, which entails the study and implementation of clinical guidelines based on organizational and system changes.

Diffusion of Innovations has been popularized by the publication of such books as Malcolm Gladwell's best seller *The Tipping Point: How Little Things Can Make a Big Difference*, in which he describes the dramatic successes and failures of business and social innovations (Gladwell, 2000). Gladwell's central argument is that a number of patterns and factors are important in virtually every influential trend of adoption, ranging from the spread of communicable diseases to the popularity of a children's television show (Glanz et al., 2008). The evidence base for diffusion in public health and health promotion has expanded in recent years. The interdisciplinary empirical review of 495 sources conducted by Greenhalgh and colleagues (2004; 2005) provides important research sources for those working in health behavior and health education. Many research-based articles have been published regarding the dissemination and adoption of physical activity programs and school-based physical education, cancer control, HIV/AIDS education and prevention programs, safer sexual practices and reproductive health, drug use, nutritional interventions, and mental health programs.

Key Concepts of Diffusion of Innovations

Diffusion of Innovations, or Diffusion Theory, describes how innovations spread through a social system through formal and information communication channels and processes (Simons-Morton, McLeroy, & Wendel, 2012). Rogers (1995, p.10) defined **diffusion** as "the process by which an innovation is communicated through certain channels over time among members of a social system." An **innovation** is "an idea, practice, or object that is perceived as new by an individual or other unit of adoption" (Rogers, 2003, p. 12). Additionally, **adoption** is "the uptake of the program or innovation by the target audience" (Glanz et al., 2008).

Many health behaviors can be considered innovations in some population groups because they have not been educated about those health behaviors or have not adopted them. Among smokers, quitting would be a possible innovation. Diffusion theory is concerned with the following key elements: (1) communication channels, (2) social system, (3) time, (4) innovation-decision process, (5) adopter categories, and (6) characteristics of the innovation. Table 9.1 provides a summary of these key elements in the Diffusion of Innovations.

Table 9.1. Summary of Key Elements - Diffusion of Innovations.

Key Element	Description
Communication Channels	Means by which information is transmitted to or within a social system
Social System	Individuals, organizations, or agencies that are potential adopters of the innovation
Time	Rate at which the innovation is diffused or the relative speed with which it is adopted
Innovation-Decision Process	Knowledge, Persuasion, Decision, Implementation, Confirmation
Adopter Categories	Innovators, Early Adopters, Early Majority, Late Majority, Laggards
Characteristics of the Innovation	Relative Advantage, Compatibility, Complexity, Trialability, Observability

Communication Channels

Communication channels are the means by which messages are spread, including mass media, interpersonal channels, and electronic communications. Innovations diffuse through a social system via two distinct communication channels: formal media and informal or interpersonal channels. Formal media sources include television, the Internet, radio, and the print media, all of which serve primarily to convey awareness knowledge. **Awareness knowledge** entails informing a large number of people about the existence and characteristics of an innovation. The second channel, informal or interpersonal channels, is the primary focus of diffusion research and theory. Those who have tried a new behavior—or, in diffusion terms, who have adopted an innovation—may discuss their opinions or subjective evaluation about the innovation with significant others who have not yet adopted the new innovation. **Subjective evaluation** includes opinions, attitudes, and beliefs about the uses and relative advantages of the innovation.

Having experience with an innovation makes an adopter a credible source of information. The attitudes of adopters about the innovation shape the attitudes and intentions of others with respect to that innovation. Those who have not yet adopted the particular innovation develop their initial impressions about it largely from talking with adopters and other potential adopters about the advantages and characteristics of the innovation. For example, if a friend or family member raves about their new computer equipment, running shoes, or gym membership, and you are in the market for such a product, you may seek to learn all that you can from their subjective evaluation of the innovation. If you were in the market for birth control, you would be interested in the experience of others who have used different types of contraceptives. If you were planning to have a mammogram for breast cancer screening, you would be interested in the experience of others who have had the procedure. Research has shown that weight loss is much more likely among those who know someone who has lost weight (Christakis & Fowler, 2007), and smokers who know someone who quit are more likely to quit than those who do not know anyone who quit smoking (Christakis & Fowler, 2008). The broader and more favorable an individual's source of information and communication channels, the more likely that individual is to adopt a new innovation or health behavior change.

Social System

We all live within different social systems that include our family, friends, coworkers, neighbors, religious and recreational groups, Internet "friends," and so on. A **social system** is a set of interrelated units that are engaged in joint problem-solving to accomplish a common goal, which includes norms and leadership (Glanz et al., 2008). Social systems are "characterized by shared beliefs and norms that define the social structures within the community and establish patterns of communication" (Simons-Morton et al., 2012, p. 185). Communication structures can be defined as formal or informal. For example, formal structures are well known to students at colleges and universities regarding formal interactions with faculty (office hours) and administrators (appointments). Informal communication structures are less standardized. For example, new students in every institution learn from upperclassmen about how to best navigate the system, take the best courses, enroll in courses with the best professors, and graduate on time. Informal communication structures are particularly important in diffusion, as they allow for the exchange of information that might not have otherwise occurred. The distinction between formal and informal structures is not always clear. As part of these formal information structures, informal information is exchanged. For example, within the formal setting of an academic classroom, the exchange of information from outside individuals may be provided informally during lectures with outside speakers.

Time

Diffusion of an innovation or a new health behavior occurs over **time**. Innovations diffuse through populations at variable rates of time, depending on a variety of different factors. Some innovations diffuse rapidly and are widespread, while others diffuse more slowly and are less extensive. Typically, adoption is quite slow at first, gains speed over time, and then trails off. This general pattern occurs regardless of the adoption, although actual periods of time involved vary considerably, as the process may play out in a matter of months, years, or decades.

Innovation-Decision Process

The process of deciding about adopting an innovation is called the **innovation-decision process**. Diffusion is a process comprising many individual decisions. Communication channels and social systems are important because they determine how information is disseminated and understood; however, individuals ultimately adopt innovations based on their perceptions of the innovation and the relative advantages of adoption. The complexity of this decision-making process influences the rate and extent of adoption. Innovations that are useful and simple to adopt often require little consideration, while useful but complex innovations often require greater consideration. Some people find something of interest to them and they quickly decide to adopt the new product or health behavior; however, others prefer to think about it for a long time as they gather information. Regardless of how long it takes, adopters go through the stages of the innovation-decision process. The length of time it takes adopters to proceed through the innovation-decision process stages is an important determinant of the diffusion rate. Rogers (2003) described the process as collecting information about the innovation to reduce uncertainty before making a commitment. The five stages of the innovation-decision process include:

- *Knowledge*—Awareness of the existence of the innovation and having practical knowledge about the underlying principles of the innovation.
- *Persuasion*—Attitudes toward the innovation, relative advantages, social norms, expected outcomes.
- *Decision*—Accepting or rejecting the innovation.
- *Implementation*—Initial adoption or trial of an innovation.
- *Confirmation*—Commitment to use, continue, or discontinue adoption of the innovation.

Note the innovation-decision process is similar to the Transtheoretical Model (TTM) and the stages of change described in Chapter 6. Both the innovation-decision process and the stages of change describe stages or processes of behavior. These stages have been applied to a wide variety of innovations and provide empirical support for the concept of behavioral change occurring in stages.

Adopter Categories

After an innovation has been widely adopted, adopters can be classified according to when they adopted the innovation. According to Simons-Morton and colleagues (2012), "based on research on the pattern of adoption of many different innovations, it turns out that all the eventual adopters, whether many or few, will tend to proportionally represent certain categories" (p. 190). Adopter categories are important for research because they not only describe the pattern and trends of adoption, but they enable health promotion planners to develop programs to target these groups. The five adopter categories include: (1) innovators, (2) early adopters, (3) early majority, (4) late majority, and (5) laggards. Figure 9.1 illustrates the bell-shaped curve for the

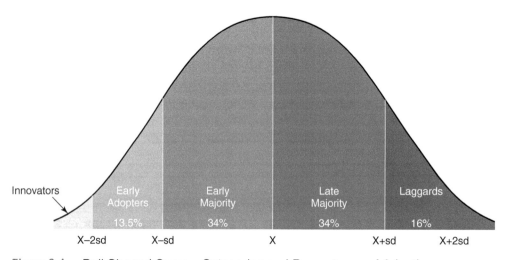

Figure 9.1.   Bell Shaped Curve—Categories and Percentages of Adoption.

http://docjourney.files.wordpress.com/2007/10/rogers-adopter-categories.jpg © Kendall Hunt Publishing Company.

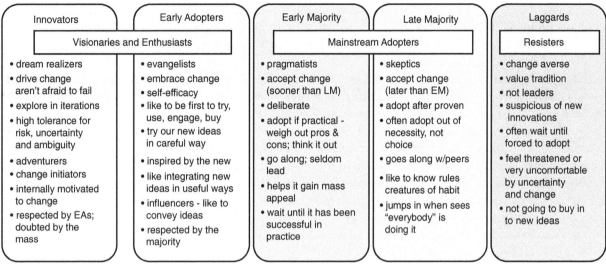

Figure 9.2. Characteristics of Adopter Categories.

© Tom Fishburne, marketoonist.com.

categories and percentages of the adoption of an innovation. Figure 9.2 presents the typical characteristics of individuals in the different adopter categories.

- **Innovators (2.5%)**—People classified as **innovators** are those individuals who are most likely to experiment with new technologies and behaviors. Innovators make up a relatively small percentage of those who adopt any particular innovation. Typically, innovators seek different types of technological outlets, which they consider, try out, and adopt or discard. Innovators comprise an important group because they seek out new information, are open to experiment with new technologies, and provide a knowledge-base for others regarding the advantages and disadvantages of innovations.

- **Early Adopters (13.5%)**—Individuals categorized as **early adopters** are those who tend to have access to a wide variety of media outlets and social networks, including access to individuals classified as innovators. Early adopters are important in the diffusion process because they represent key individuals within the community whose actions often influence the behaviors of others.

- **Early Majority (34%)**—The **early majority** represents a normative population that is innovative, but adopts after more innovative others have adopted. Typically, the early majority have standard or less access to information and are less able to adopt innovations as compared with early adopters. The early majority is an essential classification as they determine how normative an innovation can be considered. The extent of the early majority largely defines the magnitude of the diffusion of an innovation.

- **Late Majority (34%)**—The **late majority** comprises people who adopt an innovation once it is established well enough that it is normative and they have observed the benefits of the innovation by witnessing a large number of those in their social system adopt and benefit from the innovation. Typically, the late majority have limited access to sources of information and may be initially skeptical about change or adopting a particular innovation.

- **Laggards (16%)**—Those in the **laggards** category represent individuals who are potential adopters, as well as those who ultimately never adopt the innovation. Laggards tend to have limited resources, including their social network, access to information, as well as time and money. Typically, laggards comprise individuals who are most resistant to change.

Characteristics of the Innovation

Particular characteristics of an innovation determine the rate at which it will diffuse through populations. "Useful innovations with highly favorable characteristics will be immediately and broadly appealing and widely and rapidly adopted, while innovations whose characteristics are less consistently favorable, are complex or expensive and have notable downsizes will be adopted more slowly and by fewer people" (Simons-Morton et al., 2012, p. 192). Remember that an innovation may be an idea, practice/behavior, program, product/object, or policy, and it does not necessarily have to be new—it must only be perceived as new to a particular group of individuals. The innovation-decision process is largely devoted to collecting information on the characteristics of the innovation. Innovations have 12 characteristics: (1) relative advantage, (2) compatibility, (3) impact on social relations, (4) communicability, (5) reversibility, (6) risk and uncertainty level, (7) trialability, (8) complexity, (9) time, (10) commitment, (11) modifiability, and (12) observability. These 12 key determinants of diffusion's speed and extent are divided into three sections. Seven characteristics best apply to the decisions people make before they adopt the innovation (preadoption characteristics), two apply to the actual process of adoption (adoption characteristics), and three apply to the continuation or maintenance of the adoption (continuation characteristics). Table 9.2 provides a listing of the 12 attributes that are key determinants of diffusion's speed and extent.

Rogers (1995; 2003) and others (e.g., Greenhalgh et al., 2004; 2005) have comprehensively reviewed the attributes or characteristics of innovations that are most likely to affect the speed and extent of the adoption and diffusion process. The five core attributes for which a strong body of evidence exists include: (1) relative advantage, (2) compatibility, (3) complexity, (4) trialability; and (5) observability. The following paragraphs detail these five attributes which best predict diffusion's speed and extent.

Relative Advantage

Successful innovations are those that have a **relative advantage** over the alternatives and are currently available. An innovation will only be adopted if it is seen as better than the idea, product, or program it supersedes. Adoption of an innovation may involve certain resources, such as time, skills, effort, and money, and often requires giving up a current practice that competes with the new innovation (Simons-Morton et al., 2012). Therefore, there may be costs or barriers as well as advantages or benefits of adopting a particular innovation. Both actual and perceived relative advantages are important in determining adoption. An innovation has an important relative advantage if it has a positive impact on social relations. Innovations that promote

Table 9.2.   Diffusion of Innovations: Key Determinants of Speed and Extent.

I. Preadoption Characteristics

• *Relative Advantage*—Is the idea, product, or practice better than what it will replace?
• *Compatibility*—Does the innovation fit with the intended audience and/or cultural values and practices?
• *Impact on Social Relations*—Does the innovation have a disruptive effect on the social system?
• *Communicability*—Can the innovation be understood clearly and easily?
• *Reversibility*—Can the innovation be reversed or discontinued easily?
• *Risk and Uncertainty Level*—Can the product or practice be adopted with minimal risk and uncertainty?
• *Trialability*—Can the innovation be tried or practiced before making a decision to adopt?

II. Adoption Characteristics

• *Complexity*—Is the innovation easy to adopt and use?
• *Time*—Can the innovation be adopted with a minimal investment in time?

III. Continuation Characteristics

• *Commitment*—Can the innovation be used effectively with only modest commitment?
• *Modifiability*—Can the innovation be updated and modified over time?
• *Observability*—Are the results of the innovation easily evident and measurable?

social status or facilitate social interaction have great advantages over innovations that do not. For example, cell phones have been widely adopted because they have great advantages over landlines by enabling people to connect in almost any place and at any point in time. While perceived relative advantage may be sufficient for trial and implementation, actual relative advantage is necessary for continual adoption of an innovation. For example, extensive research has established the relative advantages of seat belts and air bags; however, their initial adoption was delayed because the relative advantages were not immediately evident.

Compatibility

Innovations that display **compatibility** with the intended users' sociocultural values, practices, norms, beliefs, and perceived needs are more readily adopted. In other words, innovations that are consistent with a person's current attitude and behavior and do not depart too radically from past ideas or innovations of a similar nature are more likely to be adopted. Compatibility may be considered at the individual or the organizational level. The concept of *reinvention* is often identified as a unique feature of an innovation and can be thought of as an extension of compatibility. If potential adopters can adapt, change, modify, and update an innovation to suit their own needs and context, the innovation will be adopted more easily. For example, electric toothbrushes do not depart radically from manual toothbrushes in nature; however, this innovation has been widely adopted because electric toothbrushes are more effective at removing plaque and stains, and maintaining healthy gums.

Complexity

Innovations perceived as easy to use are more likely to be adopted. Complex innovations, or those that require extensive knowledge and skill, tend to be less widely adopted and are adopted at slower rates compared to innovations that are less complex (DiClemente, Salazar, & Crosby, 2013). A key concept that applies to **complexity**, and has appeared in many other models and theories throughout this textbook, is self-efficacy. Whether the issue is to adopt the innovation or to continue the use of an innovation after its initial adoption, community members must feel confident in the use of the innovation or the performance of the innovative behavior. Self-efficacy is particularly applicable to the initial use of an innovation or the initial practice of an innovative behavior. Aerobic exercise can be considered an innovation designed to avert the onset of obesity and diabetes for those who have never exercised. People who have never engaged in aerobic exercise may not know which running shoes to purchase, what clothes to wear, where to exercise, or even how to exercise.

Trialability

Innovations that have a high degree of **trialability** at a low cost and are reversible are more likely to be adopted than innovations that require expensive and long-term commitment. People do not want to make a substantial commitment to an innovation only to find out that it does not work well or is not compatible for them. Being able to try an innovation without making a substantial commitment can resolve a great deal of uncertainty. For example, gyms frequently offer trial memberships that give people just enough time in the gym to experience some initial success, thus prompting them to consider paying for a membership. Most health-protective behaviors do have a high degree of trialability—for example, eating a low-fat diet, physical activity, condom use, smoking-cessation programs, and other programs designed to allow individuals to try healthy behaviors before committing to anything long-term.

Observability

Innovations that have a high degree of **observability**, or are easily observed by others, are more likely to be adopted than those that are not easily observable. Observability has the potential to facilitate the rate of adoption from innovators through late majority and even into the laggards. Innovations that cannot be tried prior to commitment may be more likely to be adopted if the favorable experience of others can be observed. The effect of adoption can sometimes be immediately observed, but sometimes the effects of adoption may not be readily obvious. Observation can be vicarious in the sense that one can directly observe the adopter, or the experience of adoption may be described in words, on videos, or by similar means. For example, a young female may have concerns about Gardasil® (a vaccine to help protect against infection of the human papillomavirus—HPV). It is possible for her to observe a friend receiving the vaccine and to be informed that no long-lasting pain or side effects were experienced.

Application of Diffusion of Innovations

Diffusion theory provides insight into how useful innovations are adopted and how to facilitate the adoption process. Diffusion theory is based mainly on retrospective research on the adoption of innovations and merely secondarily on research related to efforts to promote the Diffusion of Innovations. In health promotion, we are concerned with prospective approaches to increase the rate and extent of adoption of healthy behaviors. The principles of diffusion theory can be useful in planning health promotion interventions. One example involves current efforts to develop the innovation of microbicides for the purpose of decreasing the likelihood of women being infected with HIV and other sexually transmitted infections (STIs).

In the absence of a vaccine, novel biomedical methods for the prevention of HIV transmission are a public health priority. Physical barriers such as condoms have been repeatedly demonstrated to have a high efficacy in the prevention of HIV transmission and other STIs during sexual activity. Condoms, however, remain largely under the control of the male partner, and in many societies women simply cannot negotiate condom use. A female-controlled method to prevent or reduce HIV risk is highly desirable, especially if it can be used with a condom or other barrier method. Recently, vaginal microbicides, such as Carraguard, Cyanoviran, nonoxynol-9 (N9) and PRO 2000, have been developed, tested, and proven to be effective (CDC, 2018). Microbicides are chemical agents used topically by women within the vagina in order to prevent infection of HIV and potentially other sexually transmitted pathogens. Prototype microbicides are designed to be inserted prior to each act of sexual intercourse and could also be contraceptive, although most current potential microbicides are not contraceptive. In order for the innovation of a vaginal microbicide to be successful in reducing HIV transmission through being widely accepted and available, the microbicide will need to be proven effective, nontoxic, odorless, colorless, easily administered, and cheap to manufacture (Weber, Desai, & Darbyshire, 2005).

The successful use and adoption of an innovation, such as vaginal microbicides will most likely require behavioral intervention, such as education, skill acquisition, and access to the product. The adoption of this innovation will require both men and women to change longstanding practices. It has become apparent that women may want or need to include their male sexual partners in the use of microbicides (Smith & Magnet, 2007). Given this observation, an important question is: How well do vaginal microbicides align with social relations as one of the characteristics of a successful innovation? For example, researchers have rarely investigated whether or not women are willing to apply the microbicidal gel and whether men are accepting of their female partners using microbicidal gel.

When investigating vaginal microbicides according to the attributes or characteristics of innovations most likely to affect the speed and extent of the adoption and diffusion process, we can apply the five core attributes of (1) relative advantage, (2) compatibility, (3) complexity, (4) trialability, and (5) observability.

- *Relative Advantage*—The relative advantage of using a vaginal microbicide over the traditional method of HIV prevention (i.e., condom use without a vaginal microbicide) may prove to be quite substantial. Unfortunately, one of the most frequent errors in the use of microbicides is the nonuse of condoms. Vaginal microbicides are recommended in addition to using condoms. The relative advantages of vaginal microbicides have led to research to determine whether the introduction of microbicidal gel has been beneficial or not in reducing HIV and other STIs (Foss, Vickerman, Heise, & Watts, 2003; Karmon, Potts, & Getz, 2003).
- *Compatibility*—One could imagine that compatibility may be relatively low for vaginal microbicides, as women may be unwilling to apply the gel in preparation for sexual intercourse, or men may not want to have the gel applied due to lubrication issues. In some cultures women may have concerns regarding taking the initiative by introducing a vaginal microbicide to their sexual partners.
- *Complexity*—The complexity of using a vaginal microbicide may be an issue. Just as condoms and birth control pills are often used incorrectly, potential for error also exists with microbicides. Error could take

the form of applying the microbicidal gel too far in advance of sexual activity, improper storage of the microbicidal gel, using inadequate amounts of the product, using other substances in conjunction with the product, or not using a condom with the gel. It is important for users to be instructed on the proper use of the microbicidal gel without compromising its effectiveness.

- *Trialability*—Vaginal microbicides have a high degree of trialability, as they can be adopted at a low cost and are easily reversible without a long-term commitment. Health promotion educational interventions on the use and benefits of vaginal microbicides should provide samples of microbicidal gel products to participants. It is important for people to have an opportunity to first try or sample a product before making a decision to adopt the innovation.
- *Observability*—Perhaps the greatest barrier to the rapid diffusion of vaginal microbicides is the inherent lack of observability. This could be partially addressed by women and men sharing their successful experiences with friends; however, the relatively private nature of the use of microbicidal gel is likely to prohibit discourse regarding the innovation.

Given these considerations, the diffusion of the innovation of vaginal microbicides has proven to be limited. Health promotion interventions are needed to promote the relative advantages of the innovation in ways that would make it socially and practically acceptable to both men and women. A female-controlled method to prevent or reduce HIV risks has its advantages, but it also suffers from a number of barriers and disadvantages which must be overcome before widespread adoption is likely.

Summary

Diffusion of Innovations is defined as the process by which an innovation is communicated through certain channels over time among members of a social system. The principles of diffusion theory can be useful in planning health promotion intervention programs. The first section of the chapter covered the history of the Diffusion of Innovations. Also presented was a description and example of each of the key constructs of the Diffusion of Innovations: (1) communication channels, (2) social system, (3) time, (4) innovation-decision process (knowledge, persuasion, decision, implementation, confirmation), (5) adopter categories (innovators, early adopters, early majority, late majority, laggards), and (6) characteristics of the innovation (relative advantage, compatibility, complexity, trialability, observability). The last section of the chapter provided an example of the application of the Diffusion of Innovations relative to safer sexual behaviors.

References

Christakis, N. A., & Fowler, J. H. (2007). The spread of obesity in a large social network over 32 years. *New England Journal of Medicine, 357,* 370–379.

Christakis, N. A., & Fowler, J. H. (2008). The collective dynamics of smoking in a large social network. *New England Journal of Medicine, 358,* 2249–2258.

DiClemente, R. J., Salazar, L. F., & Crosby, R. A. (2013). *Health behavior theory for public health: Principles, foundations, and applications.* Burlington, MA: Jones & Bartlett Learning.

Foss, A. M., Vickerman, P. T., Heise, L., & Watts, C. H. (2003). Shifts in condom use following microbicide introduction: Should we be concerned? *AIDS, 17,* 1227–1237.

Gladwell, M. (2000). *The tipping point: How little things can make a big difference.* Boston: Little, Brown.

Glanz, K., Rimer, B. K., & Viswanath, K. (2008). *Health behavior and health education: Theory, research, and practice* (4th ed.). San Francisco: John Wiley.

Greenhalgh, T., Robert, G., Macfarlane, F., Bate, P., & Kyriakidou, O. (2004). Diffusion of Innovations in service organizations: Systematic review and recommendations. *Milbank Quarterly, 82,* 581–629.

Greenhalgh, T., Robert, G., Macfarlane, F., Bate, P., Kyriakidou, O., & Peacock, R. (2005). Storylines of research in Diffusion of Innovation: A meta-narrative approach to systematic review. *Social Science & Medicine, 61,* 417–430.

Karmon, E., Potts, M., & Getz, W. M. (2003). Microbicides and HIV: Help or hindrance? *Journal of Acquired Immune Deficiency Syndrome, 34,* 71–75.

Mosteller, F. (1981). Innovation and evaluation. *Science, 211,* 881–886.

Oldenburg, B., Sallis, J., French, M., & Owen, N. (1999). Health promotion research and the diffusion and institutionalization of interventions. *Health Education Research, 14,* 121–130.

Rogers, E. M. (1995). *Diffusion of Innovations* (4th ed.). New York: Free Press.

Rogers, E. M. (2003). *Diffusion of Innovations* (5th ed.). New York: Free Press.

Ryan, B., & Gross, N. C. (1943). The diffusion of hybrid seed corn in two Iowa communities. *Rural Sociology, 8,* 15–24.

Simons-Morton, B., McLeroy, K., & Wendel, M. (2012). *Behavior theory in health promotion practice and research.* Burlington, MA: Jones & Bartlett Learning.

Smith, R., & Magnet, S. (2007). The introduction of vaginal microbicides must also target men. *Journal of Men's Health and Gender, 4,* 81–84.

Weber, J., Desai, K., & Darbyshire, J. (2005). The development of vaginal microbicides for the prevention of HIV transmission. *PLoS Medicine, 2,* 142.

World Health Organization (WHO). (2018). *Microbicides.* Retrieved from http://www.who.int/hiv/topics/microbicides/microbicides/en.

Chapter 9—Review Questions

1. Early research on the Diffusion of Innovations was primarily conducted on agricultural products. What were the general findings of early research and how did they impact diffusion theory?

2. According to Rogers, what does the term "diffusion" mean?

3. Identify and describe the six key elements which comprise the Diffusion of Innovations.

4. Compare and contrast the two main communication channels within social systems. How is information conveyed through each of these channels? How does the type of information vary between the two channels?

5. A key component of the Diffusion of Innovations is time. What does the Diffusion of Innovations posit regarding the timeframe of innovation adoption?

6. Which construct of the Diffusion of Innovations is similar to the Transtheoretical Model (TTM)? Why?

7. Compare and contrast the five adopter categories and include the relative percentages for each category.

8. Innovations have 12 characteristics. Identify and describe which five characteristics have been backed by extensive empirical research.

9. Contemplate three of your health behaviors (physical activity, diet, sleeping habits, safety belt use, etc.) and identify which innovation characteristic persuaded you the most to adopt the health behavior.

10. This chapter applied the Diffusions of Innovations to the use of microbicides by women to reduce the incidence of HIV infection. Identify a potential health promotion program within your community which could utilize diffusion theory as a framework.

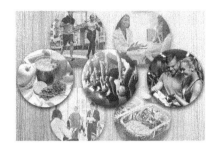

CHAPTER 10
Community Organization and Community Building

Community organizing and community building have received much attention due to the increasing focus on community-based health interventions. Community organizing and building posits that health behaviors are produced by the surrounding social context and environment. This chapter provides information on methods and processes health educators can utilize for community organizing and building. Models which were created by governmental and professional agencies for the purpose of community organizing and building are highlighted. This chapter concludes with an applied example relative to youth living in distressed environments.

History of Community Organization

According to Gavin and Cox (2001), the term "community organization" was first used by social workers in the 1800s in reference to the services they provided to immigrants and the poor. Early approaches of community organization focused on collaboration, cooperation, and consensus. These values aided communities in self-identification and problem-solving. However, a new form of community organization was developed in the 1950s. This new form of community organization, coined as "social action," encompassed confrontation and conflict as a means to facilitate social change. Social action rectified power imbalances by generating unrest and dissatisfaction within community members in order for them to identify strategies with which to bring about social change (Alinsky, 1969).

Since the 1950s, community organization has been utilized to achieve such social change objectives as civil rights, women's rights, labor rights, gay rights, and disability rights (Minkler, Wallerstein, & Wilson, 2008). Relative to public health, community organization strategies have been utilized to address the HIV/AIDS crisis and the New Right's movement was employed to ban abortion in the 1980s and 1990s. Moreover, thanks to the progress of technology, computers are now used to build online communities and organizations for virtually any health initiative (Herbert, 2004).

Another concept related to community organization is community building, which focuses on community assets and identification (Walter, 2004; Chavez, Minkler, Wallerstein, & Spencer, 2007). The practice of community building is reflected in ELEVATE, a national campaign aimed at increasing awareness about HIV/AIDS among Black women (Black Women's Health Imperative, 2012). This particular community-building project is based upon feminist organizing processes (Hyde, 1996). Although research and practice related to community building are underdeveloped, community building is gaining popularity as a complementary framework to community organization.

The Concept of Community

Understanding the concept of community is integral when discussing community organization or community building. **Community** as "a locale or domain that is characterized by the following elements: (1) membership—a sense of identity and belonging; (2) common symbol systems—similar language, rituals, and ceremonies; (3) shared values and norms; (4) mutual influence—community members have influence and are influenced by each other; (5) shared needs and commitment to meeting them; and (6) shared emotional connection—members share common history, experiences, and mutual support" (Israel, Checkoway, Schulz, & Zimmerman, 1994). Typically, a community is thought to encompass a geographic location; however, a community may also be based upon common characteristics, such as ethnicity, sexual orientation, or occupation (Fellin, 2001).

Two theories are important to the understanding of community: (1) the ecological system perspective, and (2) the social systems perspective. The **ecological system perspective** focuses on the population characteristics, surrounding physical environment, and social structure of communities, all of which are useful when studying autonomous geographical communities (Sallis, Owen, & Fisher, 2008). In contrast, the **social systems perspective** primarily focuses on the formal organization and interactions of community subsystems in relation to other community systems (Fellin, 2001). Belief communities are subsystems or units which reflect social problems within a community and enhance the structure to accommodate social, political, and economic developments and parallel the concepts of the social systems perspective.

Identifying core issues within a community influences the type of community system perspective that is appropriate. For example, Peace Corps volunteers often take on the role of community developers; in doing so they typically focus on geographical communities. In contrast, individuals who are advocates for social action believe that communities should organize around issues such as unemployment and affordable housing because of their socioeconomic consequences in local communities (Checkoway, 1989; Rinku Sen, 2003).

Community Organizing Methods

Community organization is defined as "a process through which communities are helped to identify common problems or goals, mobilize resources, and in other ways develop and implement strategies for reaching their goals they have collectively set" (Minkler, 1997). Because more attention is now focused on broadening communities, the concepts of citizen participation, grass-roots participation, community participation, macro practice, community empowerment, community development, and community capacity have become more prominent in the practice of community health education. Table 10.1 provides a definition for each of these

Table 10.1. Key Terms Associated with Community Organizing.

Term	Definition
Citizen Participation	Bottom-up mobilization of community members for the purpose of improving community conditions.
Grass-Roots Participation	Bottom-up efforts that involve collective measures of people taking actions on their own behalf based on the identification of local needs and resources.
Community Participation	Involvement of people in a community to solve problems which affect their lives.
Macro Practice	Methods that deal with problems beyond the individual, family, or small group.
Community Empowerment	The process of enabling people in communities to increase control by taking action aimed at economic, environmental, cultural, political and/or social change.
Community Development	A process where people come together to take collective action and generate sustained solutions to address community problems.
Community Capacity	The process of developing and strengthening the skills and resources that communities need to adapt, survive, and thrive in an ever-changing world.

terms. Health educators who assist in community organization work under several assumptions that were outlined by Ross (1967):

- Communities of people can develop the capacity to deal with their own problems. People want to change and can change.
- People should participate in making, adjusting, or controlling major changes taking place in their communities.
- Changes in community living that are self-imposed or self-developed have a meaning and permanence that imposed changes do not have.
- A holistic approach can deal successfully with problems with which a fragmented approach cannot cope.
- Democracy requires cooperative participation and action in the affairs of the community, and people must learn the skills which make this possible.
- Frequently, communities of people need help in organizing to deal with their needs, just as many individuals require help coping with their individual problems.

There is no one specific model to utilize when organizing a community, but rather there are many different methods. The most commonly used method was put forth by Rothman and Tropman (1987). It includes: locality development, social planning, and social action. **Locality development** is community development which seeks community-member participation to create self-initiated change. This process heavily relies upon consensus and cooperation which build a sense of community among group members. **Social planning** focuses on the problem-solving process and typically includes outside consultation. Social planning is task-oriented, whereas, locality development is process-oriented. **Social action** focuses on the redistribution of power to benefit disadvantaged persons. Social action is both task-oriented and process-oriented.

The methods created by Rothman and Tropman (1987) have been utilized for many years, but they are "problem-based and organizer-centered, rather than strength-based and community-centered" (Minkler & Wallerstein, 2002), and these become limiting factors. Minkler, Wallerstein, and Wilson (2008) created a new model which incorporates collaborative empowerment and community building. The four-quadrant model contains strength-based and needs-based on the vertical axis, and consensus and conflict on the horizontal axis. As Minkler and Wallerstein (2002) suggested, "although some organizing efforts primarily have focused in on one quadrant, the majority incorporate multiple tendencies, possibly starting as a result of a specific need or crisis and moving to a strength-based community capacity approach."

Processes of Community Organizing and Community Building

It is important for health educators to understand their role in the community organizing and building process. Health educators would normally take on a leading role in many other kinds of projects; however, as outsiders to the community, they should become facilitators and allow leaders to emerge from within the community. While there are many processes to facilitate community organizing and community building, a general model created by McKenzie, Neiger, and Smeltzer (2005) is presented below. This generic approach contains only the basic elements regarding community organizing and building. The 10 general steps are: (1) recognizing the issue, (2) gaining entry into the community, (3) organizing the people, (4) assessing the community, (5) determining the priorities and setting goals, (6) arriving at a solution and selecting intervention strategies, (7) implementing the plan, (8) evaluating the outcomes of the plan of action, (9) maintaining the outcomes in the community, and (10) looping back. Figure 10.1 illustrates a summary of the 10 general steps that can be utilized for community organizing and building.

Recognizing the Issue

Community organizing and community building begin when someone perceives an issue or an unmet need within the community. This person would be considered the initial organizer. The **initial organizer** is the individual who gets the community organizing and building process started even if they are not the primary organizer through the entire process. An initial organizer can be either a community member or a community outsider; therefore, movements are either grass-roots or top-down. A **grass-roots movement** is always initiated from within the community and is organized from the bottom up. Grass-roots movements entail "bottom-up efforts of people taking collective actions on their own behalf, and they involve the use of a sophisticated blend of confrontation and cooperation in

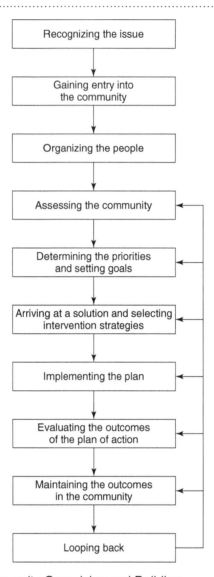

Figure 10.1. General Steps in Community Organizing and Building.

Adapted from McKenzie, J. F., Neiger, B. L., & Smeltzer, J. L. (2005). *Planning, implementing & evaluating health.*

order to achieve their needs" (Perlman, 1978). A **top-down movement** is initiated from outside the community and is organized from the outside in. Grass-roots movements tend to be more successful than top-down movements. "All historic evidence indicates that significant community development takes place when local community people are committed to investing themselves and their resources in the effort" (Kretzmann & McKnight, 1993).

Gaining Entry into the Community

Depending upon whether a community member or a community outsider has identified the problem, this second step may or may not be needed. If the issue was identified by a community member, there is no problem of gaining entry to the community because the member is already a part of the community. However, if the person who identifies the issue is a community outsider, it will be necessary to gain entry into the community. Braithwaite, Murphy, Lythcott, and Blumenthal (1989) stressed the importance of gaining entry into a community through the use of gatekeepers. **Gatekeepers** are individuals who, either formally or informally, control the "political climate" of the community. They know how the community functions and how to get tasks accomplished. Community gatekeepers include but are not limited to politicians, business leaders, education leaders, and clergy. Prior to seeking out community gatekeepers, health educators must thoroughly study the community in order to be both culturally sensitive and culturally competent. Health educators must be able to work within the cultural contexts of the community and be aware if there are any cultural differences within the community. Once the health educators have done the necessary community research, they may approach appropriate gatekeepers for assistance.

Organizing the People

The third step encompasses obtaining support from community members. It is best to recruit individuals who are interested in resolving the problem or issue. These individuals will create a core group known as the executive participants. **Executive participants** become the backbone of the community organizing and building movement and will take on the majority of the workload (Brager, Specht, & Torczyner, 1987). From this core group, a leader or coordinator with leadership skills and concern for the community will emerge. With a leader in place, the group must be expanded. Group members will be categorized as either active, occasional, or supporting participants. **Active participants** engage in the majority of group activities and are willing to put work in wherever they are needed. **Occasional participants** become a part of the group activities on an irregular basis and usually only when a big decision is being made. **Supporting participants** contribute to the group's membership numbers and resources (funding, facilities, supplies, etc.), but are rarely involved in group activities. Once the core group is expanded to include the active, occasional, and supporting participants, the entire group may be referred to as a coalition. A **coalition** is "a formal, long-term alliance among a group of individuals representing diverse organizations, factors, or constituencies within the community who agree to work together to achieve a common goal" (Butterfoss & Whitt, 2003). "Building and maintaining effective coalitions have increasingly been recognized as vital components of much effective community organizing and community building" (Minkler, 1997).

Assessing the Community

Community building "is an orientation to community that is strength based rather than need based and stresses the identification, nurturing, and celebration of community assets" (Minkler, 1997). In contrast to community organization, community building is concerned with a community assessment which focuses on the assets and capabilities of the community. To determine the needs and assets of a community, either a traditional needs assessment could be completed or a newer technique called mapping community capacity could be performed. A **needs assessment** is a process through which data relating to the community problems are collected and analyzed. Through data analysis, community problems emerge and are prioritized in order of importance, and intervention strategies are developed to deal with the problems. **Mapping community capacity** is a process which identifies the community's assets, not its problems. This is done by utilizing an actual map to identify community assets.

There are three categories of community assets, based upon their availability to the community: (1) primary building blocks, (2) secondary building blocks, and (3) potential building blocks (McKnight & Kretzmann, 1997). **Primary building blocks** are the most accessible assets; they are located within neighborhoods and are controlled by neighborhood members. **Secondary building blocks** are the next-accessible assets; they are located within neighborhoods but are primarily controlled by individuals who live outside the neighborhood. **POTENTIAL building blocks** are the least accessible assets because they are outside the neighborhood and are controlled by individuals who are also outside the neighborhood. When health educators know the needs of the community, they can utilize the available community assets to deal with the problem.

Determining Priorities and Setting Goals

Once the community's problems are identified, the community group can begin goal-setting. The goal-setting process contains two phases: (1) identifying priorities and (2) goal writing. It is necessary for the community group to identify which community problems have priority over others. Prioritizing the community's problems also helps to establish what the community group wants to accomplish. The priority list is then used to write appropriate goals. It is the responsibility of community stakeholders to set priorities and write goals to ensure that the interests of the community members are kept at the forefront. **Stakeholders** are individuals who have something to gain or lose from the community organizing and building movement

(McKenzie et al., 2005). While this process seems simple, the reality is that it takes a great facilitator to get stakeholders to agree on priorities and goals.

Arriving at a Solution and Selecting Intervention Strategies

There are multiple solutions for every community problem; however, the community group is responsible for choosing a course of action through consensus. It is important for the group to look at the advantages and disadvantages of each alternative solution, making sure to consider both the short-term and long-term effects, as well as the effects on the community, such as community acceptability and cost-effectiveness. When deciding on a solution, the group may choose one or more intervention strategies. The majority of the task of selecting appropriate intervention strategies can be delegated to subcommittees. The work done by the subcommittees will contribute to the larger plan of action. The plan of action is a formally written proposal that is provided to the community group for final approval.

Implementing, Evaluating, Maintaining, and Looping Back

The four final steps of the community organizing and building process include implementing the plan of action, evaluating the outcomes of the plan of action, maintaining the outcomes created by the plan of action, and possibly "looping back" to make any necessary amendments to the plan of action. The implementation process encompasses identifying and collecting the necessary resources for implementation, in addition to creating an implementation timeline. The evaluation process involves identifying whether the outcomes of the intervention strategies met the goals of the plan of action. Maintaining the intervention outcomes consists of determining the availability of long-term resources to sustain the plan of action. Lastly, it may be necessary for the community group to loop back and make adjustments to the plan of action to make the intervention strategies more effective.

Community Organizing and Community Building Models

Thus far, this chapter has provided a basic generic approach to community organizing and community building. There are some models, however, created by governmental agencies and professional organizations, that target specific community health problems. It is important for health educators to be aware of these models because they can be utilized for future community organizing and building efforts. The most widely known models are: Healthy Cities/Healthy Communities, Planned Approach to Community Health (PATCH), and Mobilizing for Action through Planning and Partnerships (MAPP).

Healthy Cities/Healthy Communities

Healthy Cities/Healthy Communities was initiated by the World Health Organization (WHO) and strives to create community ownership and empowerment by focusing on the values, needs, and participation of community members. This model has been implemented throughout the world and provides assistance to communities in need through consultations with health professionals. The U.S. Department of Health and Human Services (USDHHS) (1998) put forth a guide entitled *Healthy People in Healthy Communities* which provides health educators with a five-step framework to initiate and implement Healthy Cities/Healthy Communities. The five steps are provided below with brief descriptions:

- Step 1: Mobilize Key Individuals and Organizations—Identifies and organizes individuals who are interested in creating healthy change within their community.
- Step 2: Assessing Community Needs, Strengths, and Resources—Collecting and analyzing community data in order to set priorities.
- Step 3: Plan for Action—Requires the community group to create an approach to deal with the priorities set in the previous step. Also includes creating goals and objectives, selecting intervention strategies, and developing an intervention timeline.
- Step 4: Implement the Action Plan— Putting the intervention strategies into practice.
- Step 5: Track Progress and Outcomes—Requires the community group to evaluate whether the outcomes of the intervention produced the desired results as previously established by the goals and objectives.

Planned Approach to Community Health (PATCH)

PATCH was created by the Centers for Disease Control and Prevention (CDC) in 1983 to "strengthen state and local health departments' capacities to plan, implement, and evaluate community-based health promotion activities targeted toward priority health problems" (Kreuter, 1992). PATCH was created for application at the local level; however, this planning model also involves vertical collaboration within the governmental public health infrastructure (federal, state, and local levels) and horizontal collaboration at all levels (voluntary organizations, academia, and other partners). The PATCH model relies heavily upon community involvement and participation. Community members are responsible for decision-making and the majority of the workload; however, they typically receive consultative assistance from different levels, such as local health departments and the CDC. Empirically, PATCH has a "good track record for facilitating collaborative, community-based programs" (Speers, 1992). The PATCH framework includes such essential elements as organizing the community's support, participation, and leadership. Additionally, community members are responsible for choosing health priorities, intervention strategies, and evaluating the program outcomes. Figure 10.2 depicts the five phases of PATCH.

Mobilizing for Action through Planning and Partnerships (MAPP)

MAPP was created by the National Association of County and City Health Officials (NACCHO) in collaboration with the Centers for Disease Control and Prevention (CDC). MAPP was developed as an approach to improve community health and quality of life through the creation of partnerships and taking strategic action. MAPP is targeted to communities, and its goal is to provide a structured framework for planning health programs. Figure 10.4 provides the six phases of the MAPP framework:

- Phase 1: Organizing for Success and Partnership Development—Creating a core group of community members and a committee of stakeholders to guide the process. Community members provide necessary input during the decision-making process.
- Phase 2: Visioning—Allows community members to have a shared vision of the future and common values which will guide them through the entire planning process.
- Phase 3: Four MAPP Assessments—Includes four assessments: (1) community strengths assessment, (2) local public health assessment, (3) community health status assessment, and (4) forces of change assessment. This phase is one of the defining characteristics of the MAPP model.
- Phase 4: Identify Strategic Issues—Prioritization and identification of important health problems within the community.
- Phase 5: Formulate Goals and Strategies—Utilizes the prioritized health problems to create feasible goals and objectives and to select appropriate intervention strategies.
- Phase 6: Action Cycle—Creating implementation and evaluation plans.

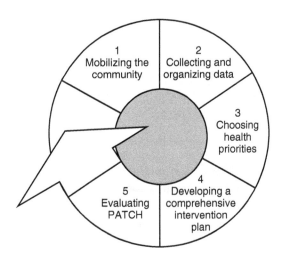

Figure 10.2.   The PATCH Model.

http://www.nap.edu/books/030908704X/xhtml/images/p20008090g408001.jpg

Application

Alcohol, substance use, fighting, bullying, and other risky behaviors are serious concerns pertaining to youth in the United States. Although risky behaviors are individual choices, they are shaped by the surrounding community and the societal context in which young people are placed. Interventions that focus on individual skill development, scare tactics, or disseminating health information are often unsuccessful because they do not address the underlying cause—namely, the risky behavioral environment. The Youth Empowerment Strategies (YES!) project provides an applied example of community organizing and community building targeted at youth living in distressed neighborhoods in California.

The Yes! Project

The YES! project was conducted from 2002 to 2005 in an effort to engage pre-adolescents as critical thinkers and problem-solvers. This three-year after school program incorporated many different community organizing and building strategies mentioned earlier in the chapter. The YES! project was funded by the CDC and utilized a strength-based approach to create empowerment. Local high school and college students were trained as facilitators to work with the youth in the afterschool program. The YES! project intervention was carried out by 37 small groups across five different schools. The groups engaged in problem-posing dialogue and other community organizing and building methods to identify community resources and strengths with which to ultimately create an action plan that addressed the community's needs (Minkler et al., 2008).

The YES! project's underlying model postulates that individuals who live in distressed neighborhoods are exposed to high levels of environmental and societal distress (Wilson et al., 2007). The high levels of exposure can lead to negative beliefs and attitudes that may decrease the prevalence of health-promoting behaviors (Wilson, Syme, Boyce, Battistich, & Selvin, 2005). The intervention model of the YES! project suggests that participation in small groups may have a positive influence on behavior. The YES! project utilized approaches designed to create a sense of community and group context in which cognitive and social skills were practiced during the decision-making process. The project participants used their skills of collaboration to facilitate group-designed social action plans which were then implemented in the surrounding neighborhoods and schools (Wilson, Minkler, Dasho, Wallerstein, & Martin, 2008). The project incorporated positive youth-development components that fostered the development of competence, confidence, connection, character, caring, and contribution to the community.

Participants

YES! program participants were fifth- and sixth-graders who attended academically underperforming elementary schools. Over the course of three years, 301 boys and girls participated in the YES! program's research component. Of the 301 boys and girls, 189 participated in the YES! program's afterschool program.

Facilitators

Local high school, college, and graduate students were selected and trained to become group facilitators. The group facilitators were critical components in the success of the social action projects. Over the course of three years, 75 group facilitators participated in 30–60 hours of training. Facilitators received either financial or course-credit compensation for their time and effort.

Curriculum

The YES! group facilitators learned various educational techniques, such as facilitating dialogue, community organizing strategies, youth development, group facilitation, cultural competence, and implementation of social action projects. The participant curriculum included group bonding, photography, photovoice, and community organizing strategies, such as school community mapping, problem selection, decision-making, strategy planning, and recruiting support (Wilson et al., 2007). After learning the basics of photography, participants took photographs which documented the qualities of their school. These photographs were placed on a group-drawn school community map. To complete the photovoice assignments, participants took photographs of the assets and problems within their school community and wrote their reflections on the photographs.

The facilitators guided group discussions regarding the underlying causes of the problems the participants perceived as prevalent in their school. The groups explored the causality of each asset and problem to create the purpose and goal for each social action project. The groups then prioritized the problems according to their perceived importance. Each group member would review the other groups' proposed social action projects. Ultimately, each group would decide on its project topic and methodology.

Social Action Projects

The YES! groups created four distinct types of social action projects: (1) awareness campaigns regarding conditions present in the school, (2) school behavior campaigns, (3) school clean-up projects, and (4) projects to improve school spirit. While these were modest projects in comparison to projects created by older youth, the participants gained a real sense of empowerment from working together to achieve their goals.

Evaluation

Questionnaires were administered to all YES! project participants after parental and student consents were obtained. Questionnaire items were adapted from published scales and included such variables as gang exposure, community violence, and peer delinquency; cognitive and attitude measures such as hope, depression, and attitudes toward violence; and additional measures of democratic awareness, belief in community action effectiveness, sense of community, leadership, and political participation and efficacy. Qualitative data were collected through year-end interviews administered by the YES! staff and school personnel. In comparison to the YES! program control group, participants in the YES! afterschool program were more likely to socialize with friends who participated in positive social behaviors and were more likely to engage in problem-solving for social problems experienced within their school. Year-end interviews illustrated that YES! program participants had a strong desire to continue to engage in social action within their schools and surrounding community.

Summary

Community organization and community building are valuable strategies to use when creating a community-based health promotion program. This chapter provided a generalized approach to community organizing and building that could be used to improve conditions within any community. Empirical research indicates that the most successful community movements are facilitated from within the community because they create a sense of ownership among the community members. In that respect, the role of a health educator becomes either facilitative or consultative when completing a community project. The Youth Empowerment Strategies (YES!) project served as an applied example of community organizing and building which targeted youth living in distressed environments. Through the use of afterschool programs, fifth- and sixth-graders gained a sense of empowerment as they tackled social problems within their schools.

References

Alinsky, S. D. (1969). *Reveille for radicals.* Chicago: University of Chicago Press.

Black Women's Health Imperative. (2012). *About ELEVATE.* Retrieved from http://www.elevateconversation.org.

Brager, G., Specht, H., & Torczyner, J. L. (1987). *Community organizing.* New York: Columbia University Press.

Braithwaite, R. L., Murphy, F., Lythcott, N., & Blumenthal, D. S. (1989). Community organization and development for health promotion within an urban Black community: A conceptual model. *Health Education, 20,* 56–60.

Butterfoss, F. D., & Whitt, M. D. (2003). Building and sustaining coalitions. In R. J. Bensley & J. Brooks-Fisher (Eds.), *Community health education methods* (2nd ed., pp. 325–356). Boston: Jones & Bartlett.

Chavez, V., Minkler, M., Wallerstein, N., & Spencer, M. (2007). *Community organizing for health and social justice.* San Francisco: Jossey-Bass.

Checkoway, B. (1989). Community participation for health promotion: Prescriptions for public policy. *Wellness perspectives: Research, theory and practice, 6,* 18–26.

Fellin, P. (2001). Understanding American communities. In J. Rothman, J. Erlich, & J. Tropman (Eds.), *Strategies of community intervention* (5th ed.). Itasca, IL: Peacock.

Garvin, C. D. & Cox, F. M. (2001). A history of community organizing since the Civil War with special reference to oppressed communities. In J. Rothman, J. Erlich, & J. Tropman (Eds.), *Strategies of community intervention* (5th ed.). Itasca, IL: Peacock.

Herbert, S. (2004). Harnessing the power of the Internet for advocacy and organizing. In M. Minkler (Ed.), *Community organizing and community building for health* (2nd ed.). New Brunswick, NJ: Rutgers University Press.

Hyde, C. (1996). A feminist response to Rothman's "The interweaving of community intervention approaches". *Journal of Community Practice, 3,* 127–145.

Israel, B. A., Checkoway, B., Schulz, A., & Zimmerman, M. (1994). Health education and community empowerment: Conceptualizing and measuring perceptions of individual, organizational, and community control. *Health Education Quarterly, 21,* 149–170.

Kretzmann, J. P., & McKnight, J. L. (1993). *Building communities from inside out: A path toward finding and mobilizing a community's assets* (Introduction) Evanston, IL: Institute for Policy Research.

Kreuter, M. W. (1992). PATCH: Its origins, basic concepts, and links to contemporary public health policy. *Journal of Health Education, 23,* 135–139.

McKenzie, J. F., Neiger, B. L., & Smeltzer, J. L. (2005). *Planning, implementing & evaluating health promotion programs: A primer* (4th ed.). San Francisco: Benjamin Cummings.

McKnight, J. L., & Kretzmann, J. P. (1997). Mapping community capacity. In M. Minkler (Ed.), *Community organizing and community building for health* (2nd ed., pp. 157–172). New Brunswick, NJ: Rutgers University Press.

Minkler, M. (1997). *Community organizing and community building for health.* New Brunswick, NJ: Rutgers University Press.

Minkler, M., & Wallerstein, N. B. (2002). Improving health through community organization and community building. In K. Glanz, B. K. Rimer, & F. M. Lewis (Eds.), *Health behavior and health education: Theory, research, and practice* (3rd ed., pp. 279–311). San Francisco: Jossey-Bass.

Minkler, M., Wallerstein, N., & Wilson, N. (2008). Improving health through community organization and community building. In K. Glanz, B. K. Rimer, & K. Viswanath (Eds.), *Health behavior and health education: Theory, research, and practice* (4th ed., pp. 287–312). San Francisco: Jossey-Bass.

National Association of County and City Health Officials (NACCHO). (2012). *MAPP framework.* Retrieved from http://www.naccho.org/topics/infrastructure/mapp/framework/index.cfm.

Perlman, J. (1978). Grassroots participation from neighborhood to nation. In S. Langton (Ed.), *Citizen partici- pation in America* (pp. 65–79). Lexington, MA: Lexington Books.

Rinku Sen, R. (2003). *Stir it up*. San Francisco: Jossey-Bass.

Ross, M. G. (1967). *Community organization: Theory, principle, and practice*. New York: Harper & Row.

Rothman, J., & Tropman, J. E. (1987). Models of community organization and macro practice perspectives: Their mixing and phasing. In F. M. Cox, J. L. Erlich, J. Rothman, & J. E. Tropman (Eds.), *Strategies of community organization: Macro practice*. Itasca, IL: Peacock.

Sallis, J. F., Owen, N., & Fisher, E. B. (2008). Ecological models of health behavior. In K. Glanz, B. K. Rimer, & K. Viswanath (Eds.), *Health behavior and health education: Theory, research, and practice* (4th ed., pp. 465–485). San Francisco: Jossey-Bass.

Speers, M. (1992). Preface. *Journal of Health Education, 23*, 132–133.

U.S. Department of Health and Human Services (USDHHS). (1998). *Healthy people in healthy communi- ties: A guide for community leaders*. Retrieved from http://odphp.osophs.dhhs.gov/pubs/healthycommunities/ hcomm2.html.

Walter, C. (2004). Community building processes. In M. Minkler (Ed.), *Community organizing and community building for health* (2nd ed.). New Brunswick, NJ: Rutgers University Press.

Wilson, N., Minkler, M., Dasho, S., Wallerstein, N., & Martin, A. C. (2008). Getting to social action: The youth empowerment strategies (YES!) project. *Health Promotion Practice, 9*, 395–403.

Wilson, N., Syme, S. L., Boyce, W. T., Battistich, V. A., & Selvin, S. (2005). Adolescent alcohol, tobacco, and mari- juana use: The influence of neighborhood disorder and hope. *American Journal of Health Promotion, 20*, 11–19.

Wilson, N., Dasho, S., Martin, A. C., Wallerstein, N., Wang, C. C., & Minkler, M. (2007). Engaging young ado- lescents in social action through photovoice: The youth empowerment strategies (YES!) project. *Journal of Early Adolescence, 27*, 1–21.

Chapter 10—Review Questions

1. Define and explain the concept of community.

2. What are the assumptions identified by Ross under which health educators work when bringing a community together to solve a problem?

3. List and describe the three community organizing methods created by Rothman and Tropman.

4. Identify and briefly describe the steps in the generalized approach to community organizing and community building presented in the chapter.

5. Explain the differences between top-down and grass-roots community organizing.

6. Define the term "gatekeeper." Identify five individuals who would be considered gatekeepers within your community.

7. Compare and contrast the differences between primary, secondary, and potential building blocks. Provide two examples for each.

8. What does the acronym PATCH stand for? What are the major components of this process?

9. What is MAPP? Identify and explain the six phases of this community approach.

10. The YES! project was an example of community organizing and community building which targeted pre-adolescent youth living in distressed environments. Provide an example of a community organizing/building program within your community. Briefly describe the purpose and goals of the project.

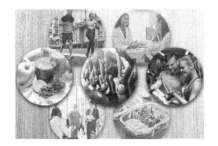

CHAPTER 11
Social Marketing

Part IV of this book emphasizes community models of health behavior: Diffusion of Innovations; Community Organization and Community Building; and Social Marketing. The community level focuses primarily on community change and building capacity to address community health problems. This chapter details social marketing, which is considered to be a framework, practice, or strategy and not a model or theory. Social marketing is concerned with employing effective marketing strategies which focus on influencing behaviors that will improve health. This chapter provides information on the key concepts of social marketing, a comparison and description of commercial marketing, and an applied example of a social marketing campaign aimed at reducing sexually transmitted infections (STIs) among young adults.

Key Concepts of Social Marketing

Social marketing has been defined as a practice, discipline, strategy, and framework, but it should never be classified as a model or theory (DiClemente, Salazar, & Crosby, 2013). Social marketing is a tool to effectively change and influence health behavior. Social marketing builds on communication theory and involves utilizing effective marketing strategies for the purpose of promoting health. It is important to emphasize that social marketing's role does not stop with people whose health behaviors are the focus; social marketing can and should target the social and physical determinants of those behaviors (Hastings & Donovan, 2002). In *Social Marketing in the 21st Century*, Anderson (2006) states that in order for social marketing to effect true social change, the focus must switch from the current downstream approach (i.e., targeting individuals) to an upstream approach (i.e., targeting structures and environmental determinants). Structures and environmental determinants include those who make decisions, such as corporate executives, government officials, legislators, media gatekeepers, community activists, lobbyists, and others who play a role in decision-making (DiClemente et al., 2013). For example, consider the public health issue of childhood obesity. It makes more sense to focus resources and efforts toward influencing school superintendents and school board members, as they are the ones who decide what meals are served in school districts and how much time is allotted for physical activity during the school day. Health professionals should use this upstream approach, which focuses on environmental factors and how they affect individual health behavior.

Kotler and Lee (2008) define **social marketing** as "a process that applies marketing principles and techniques to create, communicate, and deliver value in order to influence target audience behaviors that benefit society (public health, safety, the environment, and communities) as well as the target audience". Within this definition four key characteristics are highlighted:

- Social marketing employs traditional marketing principles, including selection of a target audience.
- Social marketing focuses on changing behavior—accepting new behaviors, modifying current behaviors, rejecting undesirable behaviors (not initiating a negative behavior), or abandoning a behavior.
- The targeted behavioral change is normally voluntary.
- The primary intended beneficiary of social marketing is society.

Social marketing is similar to commercial marketing, but there are major differences between the two. **Commercial marketing** is the sale of products and services to end-users and public and private companies.

Table 11.1.   Differences Between Social Marketing and Commercial Marketing.

Characteristic	Social Marketing	Commercial Marketing
Desired Outcome	Societal benefit	Financial gain
"Product" Sold	Positive health behavior	Goods and/or services
Perceived Competition	Current behaviors, social norms, interpersonal factors	Organizations offering similar goods and services
Targeted Behavior	Behavior causing possible physical, psychological, or financial discomfort but payoff in terms of health and societal benefit	Consumer behavior that exchanges money for a desired item/product, service, or perception

Source: Simons-Morton, B., McLeroy, K., & Wendel, M. (2012). *Behavior theory in health promotion practice and research.* Burlington, MA: Jones & Bartlett Learning.

A key difference between social marketing and commercial marketing lies in where the marketing originates (Simons-Morton, McLeroy, & Wendel, 2012). Public and private nonprofit organizations that promote public health have fewer resources to invest in social marketing campaigns than do large corporate organizations with which they compete for attention. Social marketing uses principles and techniques borrowed from commercial marketing to sell products. It is important to understand that in social marketing the term "product" refers to ideas, behaviors and health programs that are meant to enhance public health and alleviate social issues. Social marketing is used to benefit the greater good of the target population, rather than to make a profit for the marketer. Four key contrasts between social marketing and commercial marketing are highlighted in Table 11.1.

Despite the differences between social marketing and commercial marketing, a number of similarities also exist. In both social marketing and commercial marketing, customer orientation is essential and audiences are segmented to allow for more effective message tailoring. The principles of exchange lie at the core of any effective marketing strategy. These principles recognize there must be a perceived benefit to the target audience that outweighs the perceived costs such that they will engage in the desired behavior. Marketing research is used in both social and commercial marketing, and both routinely consider the "4 Ps" (product, price, place, promotion) in their strategic planning (Simons-Morton et al., 2012). These elements are described in the next sections. Figure 11.1 provides a description of the 4 Ps of social marketing.

Product

In social marketing, the **product** can be something tangible, such as an actual product (e.g., toothpaste or condoms), a program (e.g., HIV/AIDS prevention program or a smoking cessation intervention), a service (e.g., mammogram, colonoscopy, HPV vaccine, or STI screening), an intangible product such as behavioral practices (e.g., exercising or breastfeeding), or a change in attitudes, beliefs, or ideas. When designing a product, social marketers must be informed by research and can greatly enhance their efforts by using theory. It is important to understand the perceptions of the target audience regarding the health issue being addressed and also whether the product will be an adequate solution to the problem (DiClemente et al., 2013). Researchers should conduct surveys, focus groups, and interviews with the target population to better understand their perceptions regarding the particular product.

Price

The **price** of a product may be a monetary cost, such as the cost of purchasing condoms or the cost of getting a mammogram, but price can also refer to psychological or social costs. In other words, price is "what the members of the target audience must go through in order to get the product" (DiClemente et al., 2013, p. 199). Some products entail experiencing possible embarrassment (e.g., an obese individual exercising in public, going to the gas station to purchase condoms), fear (e.g., a young woman trying to negotiate condom use with her partner), physical exertion (e.g., exercise), loss of time (e.g., going to a gynecologist appointment), or even being ostracized (e.g., a smoker who tries to quit while all his friends continue to smoke). Social marketers

The Four P Components of the Marketing Mix

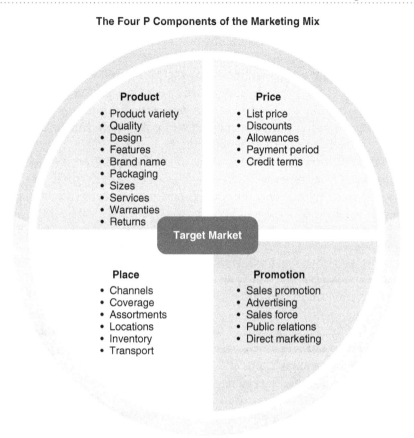

Product
- Product variety
- Quality
- Design
- Features
- Brand name
- Packaging
- Sizes
- Services
- Warranties
- Returns

Price
- List price
- Discounts
- Allowances
- Payment period
- Credit terms

Target Market

Place
- Channels
- Coverage
- Assortments
- Locations
- Inventory
- Transport

Promotion
- Sales promotion
- Advertising
- Sales force
- Public relations
- Direct marketing

Figure 11.1. The Four P's of Social Marketing.

© Kendall Hunt Publishing Company.

must figure out how to minimize costs and maximize benefits when designing products. Before deciding to buy or adopt a product, individuals consider the price and do a cost-benefit analysis to determine whether the benefits outweigh the costs.

Place

In social marketing, **place** refers to the point of contact with the target audience. Place can be thought of as the different communication channels used to get the product to the target audience. Place can be a physical location (e.g., school, health clinic, or mall), or it can be the media channels that get the product delivered to the audience (e.g., television, Internet, radio, or billboard advertisements). Thus, social marketers must consider accessibility when marketing the product. Research to inform decisions regarding place should focus on understanding the activities and habits of the target audience, as well as their experience and satisfaction with the delivery system (Weinreich, 2006). Distribution channels for the product being promoted must be chosen to maximize the convenience of the "buying" experience for the consumer. Convenience may include such things as the product's location in physical or virtual space, times when it is available, as well as the time and effort it takes to find and access the product (Glanz, Rimer, & Viswanath, 2008). For example, the placement of condom-vending machines and messages about STIs in the restrooms of nightclubs, gas stations, and college campuses increases the likelihood that the idea of safer sex, as well as the means to practice it, will be available at a convenient time and place for some consumers.

Promotion

In social marketing, **promotion** is defined as "communication strategies that inform, persuade, and influence beliefs and behaviors *relevant* to the product" (Winett, 1995, p. 347). The strategies of promotion consist of the integrated use of different communication channels, such as public service announcements (PSAs), the media, the Internet, advertising, direct mailing campaigns, editorials, promotional merchandise, interpersonal communication, or other delivery systems to promote the product. As in commercial marketing, the focus of promotion is to create demand for the product. Promotion is vital to the success of a social marketing initiative, and communication channels are a key component of the promotion element. Promotional strategies typically provide information about the other Ps, such as features of the product and the costs and benefits of adopting the product, how barriers to the product can be overcome or minimized, and where the product or service can be obtained or practiced. Almost anything goes in promotion if the message is received by the target audience, but it is important that research and theory inform the marketing strategy. Different consumer groups may respond better to one promotional strategy than to another. For example, research has shown that high-sensation-seeking adolescents may respond better to anti-marijuana messages that feature dramatic consequences of drug use rather than to messages that emphasize health statistics or social disapproval of drug use (Palmgreen, Lorch, Stephenson, Hoyle, & Donohew, 2007).

Audience Segmentation

The strengths of social marketing interventions include its cost-effectiveness, audience-driven nature, and utilization of a wide range of communication channels across a wide range of settings. Social marketing is known for its ability to alter social norms, modify a wide range of health behaviors, promote an environment of change, and empower communities (DiClemente et al., 2013). The principle of **audience segmentation** refers to "the identification of relatively homogeneous subgroups and the development of marketing strategies customized to the unique characteristics of each subgroup" (Glanz et al., 2008, p. 443). Different subgroups of the population require different marketing strategies. Subgroups value different benefits associated with a product, prioritize price considerations differently, seek and obtain product information through different channels, seek social support for behavior change differently, and respond differently to certain types of messages or other strategies.

For example, consider a marketing campaign focused on reducing sexually transmitted infections (STIs) and teenage pregnancy. Teenagers represent a diverse subgroup of the population with many different socioeconomic, cultural, and geographical characteristics. Different products and promotional strategies are necessary to meet different needs of the target population. In the 13–19 age group, some individuals are sexually active and some are not. For those who are already sexually active, educating about contraceptive use may be essential, whereas, for those who are not sexually active, encouraging continued abstinence as well as education about contraceptive use may be appropriate. Thus, an audience segmentation strategy for a campaign on reducing STIs and teenage pregnancy, based on sexual activity status, might focus on condom use for teens who are sexually active and the delay of sexual debut as well as condom use for teens who are not yet sexually active.

Social Marketing Approaches

Social marketing strategies are designed to help people make appropriate health decisions by fostering healthy and engaged communities and effective health care delivery systems supported by enlightened health policies. As early as the 1950s, the World Health Organization (WHO) pushed efforts to define health and well-being as different from a narrow disease-prevention perspective and defined health as "a state of complete mental, physical, and social well-being and not merely the absence of disease or infirmity" (WHO, 1958). Social marketing strategies must be grounded in the social, cultural, political, and economic conditions that define the current market. Not all levels of the market environment are engaged in every social marketing program, but specific social marketing approaches can be selected depending on the type of product, nature of the demand, and factors that determine behavior. We can think of these as (1) product-driven approaches, (2) consumer-driven approaches, and (3) market-driven approaches.

Product-Driven Approaches

Product-driven approaches aim to increase the product's appeal and differentiate it as positively different from the alternatives. Product differentiation is often accomplished through the social marketing practice of *branding.* In commercial marketing, branding creates a product category and associates it with desirable product attributes, such as *Crest* toothpaste, *Nike* athletic gear, *Dove* hand soap, *Banana Boat* sunscreen, and (unfortunately) *Marlboro* cigarettes. Marketers offer such products associated with a variety of benefits (e.g., good times, social status, reliable quality, good taste, and/or environmental protection). Consumers expect such benefits and continue to return to the same products in anticipation of predictable outcomes.

Consumer-Driven Approaches

Consumer-driven approaches "go beyond simply marketing the product to building demand for the product, so that maintaining behavioral momentum shifts from the marketing organization to consumers" (Glanz et al., 2008, p. 445). These approaches may be more sustainable over time than product-driven approaches, due to the nonprofit nature of social marketing. One strategy for achieving and sustaining consumer demand is to target social norms (Haines, 1998; Linkenbach, 1999). This approach is based on the theory that a great deal of behavior is influenced by perceptions of what is "normal" and the perceived rewards which result from complying with these norms (Cialdini & Goldstein, 2004). Unfortunately, the misperception of norms is common, even among peers. This is especially the case when behaviors are less publicly visible, such as taboo or illegal behaviors like sex or drug use. Perception usually trumps reality, so if a teenager believes the majority of his or her peers smoke cigarettes, then he or she is more likely to try smoking. Moreover, if a teenager thinks his or her friends are engaging in sexual activity, then they are more likely to engage in that behavior as well. Social norms marketing can be used to inform individuals about the actual frequency of behaviors among peer groups in order to create a factual perception of reality.

Market-Driven Approaches

Market-driven approaches are an extension of consumer-driven approaches. **Market-driven approaches** take options into consideration, where behavioral choices are made in light of other possibilities, many of which have their own perceived benefits. A market-driven approach must position its product as an attractive alternative to the competition. For example, social marketing for responsible drinking must provide viable alternatives, such as a designated driver, Uber, Lyft, or taxi services. The Ad Council is a significant producer of social marketing campaigns in the United States, primarily through public service announcements (PSAs). In 1983, the U.S. Department of Transportation and the Ad Council launched a market-driven approach for a drunk-driving prevention campaign branded *Friends Don't Let Friends Drive Drunk*. The mission of the campaign was to use the power of advertising to raise awareness and stimulate action against drinking and driving. The campaign featured a variety of messages aimed at increasing the severity of drunk driving, the risk of being considered a bad friend, and some specific behaviors to reduce this risk. The *Friends Don't Let Friends Drive Drunk* campaign has taken many forms, and the Ad Council has produced PSAs for television, radio, print, and online media outlets. According to the National Highway Traffic Safety Administration (NHTSA), 84% of Americans recall having seen or heard a *Friends Don't Let Friends Drive Drunk* PSA. Nearly 80% of Americans reported they took action to prevent a friend or loved one from driving drunk, and 25% indicated they stopped drinking and driving as a result of the campaign (NHTSA, 2012). Figure 11.2 illustrates an advertisement for the *Friends Don't Let Friends Drive Drunk* social marketing campaign.

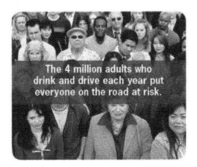

Figure 11.2.   Social Marketing Campaign: Friends Don't Let Friends Drive Drunk.

Courtesy of the Centers for Disease Control and Prevention (CDC).

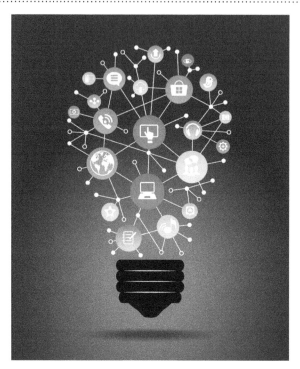

Figure 11.3. Social Media outlets for Marketing.

© Shutterstock.com.

Application of Social Marketing

Social marketing has been applied to target a variety of health behaviors, including injury prevention, environmental protection, community building, and specific health behaviors (e.g., obesity prevention, exercise, smoking cessation and prevention, heart disease prevention, breast cancer screening, family planning, reproductive health, HIV/AIDS, violence prevention). A variety of public and private sector organizations have used social marketing to target behaviors central to health promotion. Health communication can occur through large-scale campaigns, as previously described, but it is also seen in doctor-patient relationships, health education, and more broadly through newer technologies, such as the Internet, Facebook, and Twitter. Figure 11.3 illustrates some of the communication channels and technologies through which a great deal of social marketing occurs.

Winett (1995) delineated the different theoretical models that are relevant to each of the four marketing elements (4 Ps) of social marketing. These are presented in Table 11.2 and provide a guide for social marketers to select a theory that can inform each element.

- *Product*—When designing a new product, Diffusion of Innovations (Chapter 9) suggests that the marketer should consider characteristics such as relative advantage (the product is seen as better than the idea, product, or program it supersedes), compatibility (the product is suitable for existing cultural values and norms), complexity (the product is easy to use), trialability (the product is available to adopt at minimal cost or commitment), and observability (the product or innovation is able to be easily witnessed by others). From the Transtheoretical Model and Stages of Change (Chapter 6), social marketers must consider how to match product characteristics to the different stages of the target audience. For example, potential adopters in the precontemplation or the contemplation stage will view product characteristics differently than audience members who are in the action stage.
- *Price*—When considering the price of the product, we can refer back to Social Cognitive Theory (Chapter 7). One central component of Social Cognitive Theory is reinforcement. Designing a product that will reinforce its use will result in a better cost-benefit ratio. For example, rather than having the ultimate goal behavior (such as running a marathon) as the product, breaking the behavior down into smaller successive goals (such as walking a mile, then three miles, then running three miles, etc.) will increase the rate of adoption of the product. Self-efficacy also should be considered when addressing

Table 11.2. Social Marketing Variables: Relevant Theories, Models, and Frameworks.

Variable	Theory-Model-Framework	Principles	Concepts
Product	Diffusion of Innovations	Product Design	Relative Advantage, Compatibility, Complexity, Trialability, Observability
	Transtheoretical Model/Stages of Change	Matching	Precontemplation, Contemplation, Preparation, Action, Maintenance
Price	Health Belief Model	Self-Efficacy	Benefits and Barriers
	Social Cognitive Theory	Reinforcements	Feedback and Goal Setting
Place	Social Ecological Perspective	Environmental Design	Intrapersonal, Interpersonal, Organizational, Cultural, Public Policy, Physical Environment, Community
Promotion	Health Belief Model	Perception of Product	Perceived Susceptibility, Perceived Severity, Perceived Benefits, Perceived Barriers, Cues to Action, Self-Efficacy
	Theory of Reasoned Action/Theory of Planned Behavior	Cognition and Behavior	Attitude + Subjective Norms + (Perceived Behavioral Control) = Intention $\longrightarrow$ Behavior

price. If members of the target audience perceive low confidence in performing a health behavior or adopting a product, they will be less likely to adopt that particular product or behavior. Expectancy value theories, such as the Health Belief Model (Chapter 4), also play a role. The Health Belief Model components of perceived benefits and perceived barriers are directly related to how social marketers must balance the costs and benefits associated with the price of adoption.

- *Place*—When considering the place of an innovation, the Social Ecological Perspective (Chapter 4) should be considered. The importance of place was discussed by Maibach, Abroms, and Marosits (2007), who explain the social marketing perspective in terms of a social ecological framework that situates audiences and choices within geographical, economic, and cultural spaces that determine access to and value of the product. This requires a thorough understanding of intrapersonal factors (e.g., self-efficacy, motivations, demographic characteristics, skill levels, attitudes, behavior), interpersonal factors (social relationships), as well as organizational, cultural, public policy, environmental, and community factors or the characteristics of the place where decisions are made (media factors, availability of products and services, physical features of the environment, social structures, laws and regulations).
- *Promotion*—Expectancy value theories, such as the Health Belief Model (Chapter 4) and the Theory of Reasoned Action and the Theory of Planned Behavior (Chapter 5), can inform the promotion of an innovation. These theories suggest that the social marketer must create a sense of vulnerability or perceived threat surrounding the health issue through appropriate communication channels. In the Health Belief Model, creating a sense of vulnerability or threat represents the concepts of perceived susceptibility and perceived severity. It is also essential to portray the use of the product as resulting in more benefits or value than costs. This represents the concepts of perceived benefits and perceived barriers. Additionally, a reason for adhering to the message should be provided, such as "doctors recommend" or "your loved ones would want you to." In the Health Belief Model, such messages are referred to as cues to action. According to the Theory of Reasoned Action and the Theory of Planned Behavior, social marketers must promote the product according to attitudes and social norms in order to create a strong desire or intention to perform the new health behavior (e.g., working out at the gym) or obtaining a new product (e.g., an electric toothbrush).

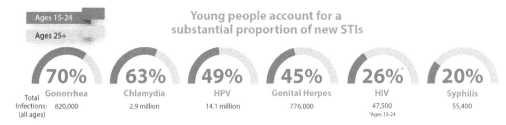

Figure 11.4.   STI Statistics in the United States.

© Kendall Hunt Publishing Company.

Applied Example

An example using the marking mix (4 Ps) strategy for a campaign to reduce STIs among young adults is illustrated in Figure 11.4.

- *Product*—The product in this marketing campaign is a set of behaviors: getting the target audience (young adults 15–24 years of age) to use contraceptives every time they have sex as well as getting the target audience to get tested for STIs.
- *Price*—The price of engaging in these behaviors includes comparing the costs (e.g., potential discomfort of negotiating condom use, cost of condoms, loss of pleasure, accessibility of a health clinic, cost of getting tested for STIs, potential distress of finding out one has an STI) to the benefits (e.g., knowing STI status, reducing risk of STIs and unintended pregnancy).
- *Place*—The place that would be designed to change behaviors might be print ads posted on college campuses, Internet websites, billboards, or local health clinics.
- *Promotion*—Promotion could be conducted through PSAs on the Internet, television, radio, billboards, media events, college campuses, and/or other community outreach venues.

Each element of the marketing mix should be taken into consideration as the program is developed, and attention should be paid to how they are all interconnected. Research and theory are necessary to shape the final product, price, place, and promotion-related decisions. Social marketing draws our attention beyond individual behavior change and toward ways that communication can affect market structure itself through policy change (e.g., fluoridation of water and iodization of salt), legislative (e.g., seat belt use), and social norms (e.g., stigma of tobacco use and obesity) to facilitate positive health behaviors.

Summary

This chapter details social marketing, which is considered a framework, practice, or strategy and not a model or theory. Social marketing is concerned with employing effective marketing strategies which focus on influencing behaviors that will improve health status. The social marketing approach utilizes the 4 Ps marketing mix: (1) product, (2) price, (3) place, and (4) promotion. The principles of social marketing contain similarities to, as well as differences from, the principles of commercial marketing. Social marketing is relevant to other theories, models, and frameworks including the Social Ecological Perspective, The Health Belief Model, Theory of Reasoned Action/Theory of Planned Behavior, Transtheoretical Model/Stages of Change, Social Cognitive Theory, and Diffusion of Innovations. Social marketing has been useful in planning health promotion intervention programs. This chapter concluded with an applied example of a social marketing campaign produced by the federal government to reduce STIs among young adults.

References

Anderson, A. R. (2006). *Social marketing in the 21st century*. Thousand Oaks, CA: Sage.

Cialdini, R. B., & Goldstein, N. J. (2004). Social influence: Compliance and conformity. *Annual Review of Psychology, 55*, 591–621.

DiClemente, R. J., Salazar, L. F., & Crosby, R. A. (2013). *Health behavior theory for public health: Principles, foundations, and applications*. Burlington, MA: Jones & Bartlett Learning.

Glanz, K., Rimer, B. K., & Viswanath, K. (2008). *Health behavior and health education: Theory, research, and practice* (4th ed.). San Francisco: John Wiley.

Haines, M. P. (1998). Social norms: A wellness model for health promotion in higher education. *Wellness Management, 14*, 1–8.

Hastings, F., & Donovan, R. J. (2002). International initiatives: Introduction and overview. *Social Marketing Quarterly, 8*, 3–5.

Kotler, P., & Lee, N. R. (2008). *Social marketing: Influencing behaviors for good*. Thousand Oaks, CA: Sage.

Linkenbach, J. W. (1999). Application of social norms marketing to a variety of health issues. *Wellness Management, 15* [entire issue].

Maibach, E., Abroms, L. & Marosits, M. (2007). Communication and marketing as tools to cultivate the public's health: A proposed "People and Places" framework. *BMC Public Health, 7*(88). Retrieved from
 http://www.biomedcentral.com/1471-2458/7/88.

National Highway Traffic Safety Administration (NHTSA). (2012). *Introduction: What is a designated driver program?* Retrieved from http://www.nhtsa.gov/people/injury/alcohol/designateddriver.

Palmgreen, P., Lorch, E. P., Stephenson, M. T., Hoyle, R. H., & Donohew, L. (2007). Effects of the Office of National Drug Control Policy's marijuana initiative campaign on high-sensation-seeking adolescents. *American Journal of Public Health, 97*, 1644–1649.

Simons-Morton, B., McLeroy, K., & Wendel, M. (2012). *Behavior theory in health promotion practice and research*. Burlington, MA: Jones & Bartlett Learning.

Weinreich, N. K. (2006). *What is social marketing?* Weinreich Communications. Retrieved from http://www .social-marketing.com/Whatis.html.

Winett, R. A. (1995). A framework for health promotion and disease prevention programs. *American Psychologist, 50*, 341–350.

World Health Organization (WHO). (1958). *The first ten years of WHO*. Geneva: World Health Organization.

Chapter 11—Review Questions

1. According to *Social Marketing in the 21st Century* by Anderson, what is the most effective way to achieve social marketing success?

2. Define social marketing. Explain the four key characteristics of social marketing.

3. Compare and contrast the differences between social marketing and commercial marketing.

4. Describe the 4 Ps of social marketing. Provide an example related to health promotion for each.

5. Identify the strengths associated with social marketing interventions.

6. Explain the principle of audience segmentation. How does this principle impact the effectiveness of health-related marketing campaigns?

7. What is the product-driven approach to social marketing? What implications does it have for the promotion of healthy behaviors?

8. What are some negative consequences of the consumer-driven approach to social marketing?

9. Market-driven approaches to social marketing are an extension of consumer-driven approaches. What extensions does this approach provide?

10. Reflect on your community. What health-related social marketing efforts are currently present? Identify one health-related campaign and discuss its purpose, goals, and target audience.

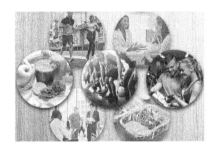

CHAPTER 12
PRECEDE-PROCEED Model

Part V of this textbook highlights the application and evaluation of theory-based interventions within the profession of health education. These final chapters focus on: PRECEDE-PROCEED Model; Measurement and Instrumentation; Design, Sampling, and Evaluation; and Future Trends and Technology in Health Education. It is imperative for health educators to apply health behavior theories when creating a health promotion program. The PRECEDE-PROCEED planning model assists program planners in effectively integrating theoretical frameworks into the foundation of programs. This chapter will present information relative to the history of the PRECEDE-PROCEED model, phases of the model, and an applied example of the model utilized within a media campaign aimed at increasing mental health literacy.

History of the PRECEDE-PROCEED Model (PPM)

A crucial skill required for program planners to design effective health promotion programs is the ability to apply health behavior theories to address health concerns among a target population. The **PRECEDE-PROCEED Model** (PPM) is a planning model which can assist program planners to incorporate theory into the programs they create. The PPM is the most widely used program-planning tool. Gielen and colleagues described the PPM as a road map that provides program planners with many alternative avenues, whereas, health behavior theories provide the proper direction to achieve the desired outcomes of the program (Gielen, McDonald, Gary, & Bone, 2008).

The PPM, as it is known currently, had its beginnings in the 1970s, when Green and colleagues created the PRECEDE framework (Green, Kreuter, Deeds, & Partridge, 1980). PRECEDE is an acronym which stands for: Predisposing, Reinforcing, and Enabling Constructs in Educational/Environmental Diagnosis and Evaluation. This initial framework addressed the need to conduct an educational diagnosis prior to implementing a program. Previously, the profession of health education had been focused on implementing programs rather than creating strategically planned programs that met the needs of the target population (Bartholomew, Parcel, Kok, & Gottlieb, 2001). The introduction of the PRECEDE framework addressed the lack of needs assessment within the profession.

PROCEED was added to the PRECEDE framework in 1991 to address the influence environmental factors exert on health and health behaviors (Gielen et al., 2008). PROCEED is an acronym which stands for: Policy, Regulatory, and Organizational Constructs in Educational and Environmental Development. Originally, the PPM contained nine phases; however, after receiving feedback from the professional community, Green and Kreuter amended the model in 2005 to reflect the current practice of health education (Gilmore, 2012).

More specifically, Green and Kreuter revised the model to include: (1) an ecological and participatory approach, and (2) accommodate new research in the field of genetics as the profession of public health has evolved to encompass these perspectives, instead of just focusing on health behavior change programs (Institute of Medicine, 2001; 2003). The 2005 revision of the PPM offered more efficient planning phases by merging the epidemiological, behavioral, and environmental assessment phases into a single phase (Epidemiological Assessment), thus making the PPM an eight-phase planning model (Gilmore, 2012).

Phases of the PRECEDE-PROCEED Model

The PPM phases focus on concepts central to the profession of health education and health promotion: (I) planning, (II) implementing, and (III) evaluating. The collaboration of these concepts within the PPM is depicted in Figure 12.1. The PPM contains eight phases (four planning, one implementation, and three evaluation). These include: (1) Social Assessment, (2) Epidemiological Assessment, (3) Educational and Ecological Assessment, (4) Administrative and Policy Assessment and Intervention Alignment, (5) Implementation, (6) Process Evaluation, (7) Impact Evaluation, and (8) Outcome Evaluation. Figure 12.2 illustrates the PPM currently utilized in practice.

Phase 1: Social Assessment

Green and Kreuter (2005) defined **social assessment** as the "application, through broad participation, of multiple sources of information, both objective and subjective, designed to expand the mutual understanding of people regarding their aspirations for the common good." During this phase, program planners conduct various data-collection activities, such as interviews, focus groups, or surveys, within the target population in order to uncover the needs of the community. When program planners collect data first-hand, they obtain what is considered to be **primary data**. Examples of primary data include surveys, focus groups, interviews, and observational study. In addition to establishing the needs of the community, a social assessment provides planners with information regarding a community's problem-solving capacity, readily available resources, and strengths. Planners should make sure they focus on the strengths of the community, as this will allow them to form more meaningful and sustained partnerships with key gatekeepers within the community (Bartholomew, Parcel, Kok, & Gottlieb, 2006). Typically, programs are predetermined in the sense that planners will have an ideal target population or health issue in mind; however, planners should elicit the participation of the community in determining other health concerns that may be important to the members of the community. It is suggested that program planners or health educators establish a planning committee, conduct community forums, and hold focus groups to encourage community participation in the health promotion program (Gielen et al., 2008).

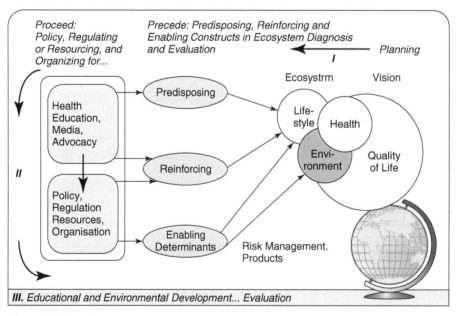

Figure 12.1.   Concepts of the PRECEDE-PROCEED Model.

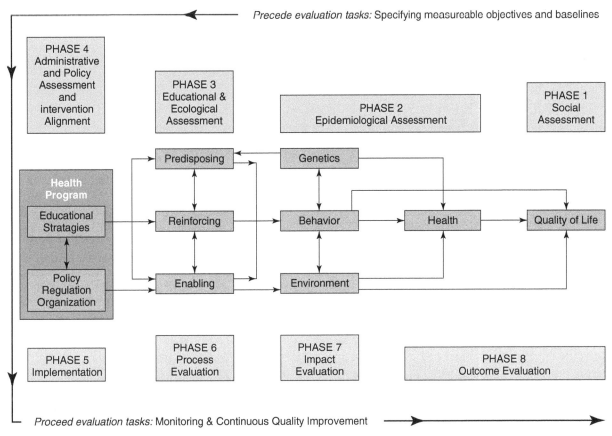

Figure 12.2.   PRECEDE-PROCEED Model.

When program planners or health educators work within a community, it is imperative for them to understand their position within the process. Program planners facilitate and lead the process of change within the community; however, they must allow leaders from within the community to emerge in order to create a sustainable partnership. Empirical evidence suggests that the most successful community programs begin within a community and lead to the cultivation of ownership among community members (Kretzmann & McKnight, 1993).

Phase 2: Epidemiological Assessment

The needs assessment is conducted during phase two and addresses health issues relative to their behavioral and environmental determinants. **Epidemiological assessment** is responsible for identifying the health problem or issue the program will address, revealing the behavioral and environmental factors that influence the health problem or issue, and transcribing the information into a set of measurable objectives for the program to utilize (Green & Kreuter, 2005). During this phase, program planners may review secondary data. **Secondary data** are data which have previously been collected by other researchers, such as vital statistics and state or national health surveys. Once the planner identifies the specific objectives the health promotion program will address, the behavioral and environmental determinants associated with the objectives can be identified (Simons-Morton, McLeroy, & Wendel, 2012).

Behavioral determinants of health issues exist on many levels. Behaviors which contribute to the presence and severity of health problems (e.g., smoking, poor nutrition, and sedentary lifestyle) are considered most proximal; whereas the behavior of individuals who can influence the actions of the person at risk (e.g., parents, spouses, and friends) are considered more distal. The third level of behavioral determinants encompass the actions of policymakers whose decisions affect the social or physical environment of the individual at risk (e.g., policy or law makers). Environmental determinants of health are external factors that are beyond the control of an individual, such as social and physical factors. Environmental factors have the potential to influence and modify health outcomes (Gielen et al., 2008).

	More Important	Less Important
More Changeable	High Priority for Program (Quadrant 1)	Low Priority for Program (Quadrant 3)
Less Changeable	Priority for Innovative Program; Evaluation Crucial (Quadrant 2)	No Program (Quadrant 4)

Figure 12.3. Prioritization Matrix.

Green, L. W., & Kreuter, M. W. (1999). Health program planning: An educational and ecological approach (3rd ed.). Mountain View, CA: Mayfield.

Once the behavioral and environmental determinants are identified, planners must then prioritize the determinants. A **prioritization matrix** is a tool which program planners may utilize to help prioritize the behavioral and environmental determinants. Figure 12.3 provides an example of a prioritization matrix. Planners prioritize factors based upon the importance and changeability of the behavioral or environmental factor. If a health problem requires immediate attention (i.e., is more important) and planners have the means to address the problem easily (i.e., it is more changeable), a program should be created to address the problem (Quadrant 1). However, if the problem does not need immediate attention (i.e., is less important) and planners lack the resources to address the problem thoroughly (i.e., it is less changeable), it may not be wise to create a program for that particular health problem (Quadrant 4). If a health determinant falls within Quadrants 2 or 3, the planner may elect to gain feedback from the community to discover their desires and the available resources to create a program to address the identified health problem.

Once the behavioral and environmental factors are selected, planners should utilize the literature as a guide to identify a theory to use as the program foundation. When considering individual behavioral change (e.g., physical activity, proper nutrition, smoking cessation, and contraceptive use), intrapersonal theories, such as the Health Belief Model (HBM) (Chapter 4), the Theory of Reasoned Action/Theory of Planned Behavior (TRA/TPB) (Chapter 5), and the Transtheoretical Model (TTM)/Stages of Change (Chapter 6) would be useful. For example, a diabetes educator may be interested in whether the HBM can predict a diabetic's adherence to a new diet. The diabetes educator could develop a nutritional intervention to teach newly diagnosed diabetics how to create balanced meals in order to control their blood sugar. Next, the diabetes educator may create a pre- and post-test survey which includes items that measure the constructs of the HBM relative to diabetes management. Based upon the survey results and data analysis, the diabetes educator could determine if any of the HBM constructs were predictive of diet adherence.

If planners want to incorporate an ecological perspective that focuses on the interaction between the individual and the environment (e.g., reducing low birth weight, gang violence, and teenage pregnancy rates) interpersonal theories, such as the Social Cognitive Theory (SCT) (Chapter 7) and various social network or social support theories (Chapter 8), would provide a comprehensive evaluation of how environmental factors impact an individual's decisions. Lastly, if a program planner or health educator intends to focus on community and organizational change (e.g., smoking bans, healthy food options for school cafeterias, requiring physical activity classes in schools), theories which motivate social action, such as Diffusion of Innovations (Chapter 9), community organization and community building theories (Chapter 10), and Social Marketing (Chapter 11) would serve as the best guide to effectively create change on an administrative or policy level.

Phase 3: Educational and Ecological Assessment

After identifying and selecting the behavioral and environmental determinants, planners must conduct an **educational and ecological assessment** which identifies and classifies factors into predisposing, reinforcing, and enabling factors that influence the likelihood of behavioral and environmental change (McKenzie, Neiger, & Smeltzer, 2005). **Predisposing factors** are "antecedents to behavior that provide the rationale or motivation for the behavior" (Green & Kreuter, 2005). More specifically, predisposing factors include an individual's awareness, attitudes, beliefs, and knowledge. For example, an individual who believes that smoking tobacco from a hookah pipe is not harmful and poses no threat to health is more likely to participate in that negative health behavior. **Reinforcing factors** are "those factors following a behavior that provide continuing reward or incentive for the persistence or repetition of the behavior" (Green & Kreuter, 2005). Examples of reinforcing factors include encouragement from family members, friends, teachers, coaches, peers, and significant others. For example, a parent might foster good nutritional practices by rewarding their child with an after dinner bike ride if the child eats all of their vegetables at dinner. **Enabling factors** are "antecedents to behavioral or environmental change that allow a motivation or environmental policy to be realized" (Green & Kreuter, 2005). Enabling factors include programs, resources, and services that assist individuals in building new skill sets which are conducive to behavior change. For example, free stress management courses offered in a workplace could provide relief to workers who are trying to quit using tobacco.

When planners try to tackle the predisposing, reinforcing, and enabling factors, they may use a combination of intrapersonal, interpersonal, organizational, or community behavior theories. Intrapersonal theories will provide the most assistance when addressing predisposing factors (Chapters 4–6). Reinforcing factors are best addressed by utilizing interpersonal theories (Chapters 7–8). Lastly, organizational and community theories are most appropriate for addressing enabling factors (Chapters 9–11).

Phase 4: Administrative and Policy Assessment and Intervention Alignment

The purpose of conducting an **administrative and policy assessment** is to determine whether the necessary capabilities and resources are available to create and implement the program (McKenzie et al., 2005). During this phase, program planners are responsible for selecting intervention strategies that match the previously identified determinants. To accomplish this, planners must align the assessments of determinants with the proper intervention strategies on two levels (Green & Kreuter, 2005). They must address the macro level first. It is imperative to consider the effect environmental and organizational systems have on the desired outcomes of the program. Second, program planners must consider the micro level. The micro level focuses on individuals, family members, friends, and peers. Intervention strategies implemented at the micro level are aimed at changing predisposing, reinforcing, and enabling factors. There are many strategies from which planners may choose. The best strategies are those that fit the context of the program, the needs of the target population, and the diagnosis discovered by the PPM. Table 12.1 provides a list of the types of intervention strategies planners or health educators may utilize within a program.

Phase 5: Implementation

Implementation is "the act of converting planning, goals, and objectives into action through administrative structure, management activities, policies, procedures, regulations, and organizational actions of new programs" (Timmreck, 1997, p. 328). When a program planner reaches this phase, the program should be finalized and ready to be put into action. It is important for planners or health educators to formulate an action plan for data collection so as to continue with the next phases of the PPM.

Table 12.1.   Types of Intervention Strategies

1.   Health communication strategies
2.   Health education strategies
3.   Health policy/enforcement strategies
4.   Health engineering strategies
5.   Health-related community service strategies
6.   Community mobilization strategies
7.   Other strategies

Source: McKenzie, J. F., Neiger, B. L., & Smeltzer, J. L. (2005). *Planning, implementing & evaluating health promotion programs* (4th ed., pp. 179–180). San Francisco: Pearson Education.

Phases 6–8: (6) Process Evaluation, (7) Impact Evaluation, and (8) Outcome Evaluation

The last three phases of the PPM are related to evaluating the program. The purpose of a **process evaluation** is to assess the extent to which the program was implemented according to the set protocol. An **impact evaluation** assesses the extent of change in the predisposing, reinforcing, and enabling factors in addition to the behavioral and environmental factors. The **outcome evaluation** assesses the effectiveness of the program and whether the program reached its goals and objectives. Process, impact, and outcome evaluation are all thoroughly addressed in Chapter 15.

Application of the PRECEDE-PROCEED Model

In 2001, the Compass Strategy was implemented in selected regions of Victoria, Australia (Wright, Mcgorry, Harris, Jorm, & Pennell, 2006). The Compass Strategy was concerned with early detection and treatment of mental disorders among adolescents. This program aimed to achieve its goal by increasing mental health literacy among adolescents and parents. Two adjacent regions of Victoria were chosen as the intervention group for the Compass Strategy. These two areas, Melbourne and Barwon, provided researchers with geographic and demographic variability. Adjoining regional areas were selected to be the comparison group used during the impact evaluation (Phase 7). The following is a summary of how the PRECEDE-PROCEED Model was utilized to create, implement, and evaluate the Compass Strategy.

Phases 1 & 2: Social and Epidemiological Assessments

The researchers utilized focus groups composed of adolescents and parents who were affected by mental health disorders to generate ideas regarding appropriate media messages that stressed the importance of early detection and treatment. Prior to beginning the intervention, the researchers conducted randomized telephone interviews with adolescents (600 from the intervention group and 600 from the comparison group) between the ages of 12 and 25. During the interview, participants were read scenarios of individuals with mental disorders and were asked to identify the specific disorder, treatments for the disorder, and possible outcomes of the disorder. The researchers performed a follow-up and repeated the telephone interviews 14 months after the intervention was implemented.

Typically, during the initial phases of the PPM, health educators examine quality of life indicators within a community to identify target populations and prominent health issues. In the Compass Strategy, researchers were able to identify key stakeholders, such as general practitioners, community health services, youth and welfare services, and consumers of mental health services, who had an interest in the mental health status of adolescents.

From the focus groups and telephone interviews, researchers were able to identify the target behavioral and environmental determinants. The focus group responses indicated that the process of early detection and treatment of mental disorders comprised four steps: (1) recognizing the problem, (2) seeking professional help for the problem, (3) receiving appropriate treatment for the problem, and (4) complying with the treatment regimen. Researchers identified social support, social norms regarding mental illness, social network connections, and mental illness stigma to be the environmental determinants relative to early detection and treatment of mental disorders.

Phases 3 & 4: Educational and Ecological Assessment and Administrative and Policy Assessment and Intervention Alignment

After identifying the behavioral and environmental determinants, researchers were able to assess the predisposing, reinforcing, and enabling factors. Predisposing factors, such as knowledge, attitudes, and beliefs all have an impact upon current health behaviors. Responses from the focus groups and telephone interviews revealed that the prominent predisposing factors among adolescents were inadequate or limited knowledge and awareness of the signs, symptoms, and severity of mental disorders, limited knowledge of treatment options for mental illness, low perceived susceptibility to mental disorders, and fear of the stigma commonly associated with mental disorders.

The focus groups and telephone interviews identified family members and friends as the most important reinforcing factor regarding social support and seeking help for mental illness. These reinforcing factors were followed by teachers, counselors, and church officials. Participant responses also indicated that their sources of social support often struggle with identifying the signs and symptoms of mental illness. Lack of resources that provide information about mental illness and how to seek treatment was assessed to be a barrier for enabling factors. Providing adequate information relative to symptoms of mental illness and sources of help was the primary enabling factor. Creating programs or services which developed skills in early detection and seeking help for mental disorders was determined to be a secondary enabling factor.

The researchers conducted an administrative and policy assessment which analyzed the available resources and policies that would either hinder or facilitate the success of the Compass Strategy. It was determined the necessary resources were available to implement and successfully evaluate the program. Researchers were provided with grant funding from the Australian government's new mental health policy, which focused on early intervention and promoting mental wellness (Australian Health Ministers, 1998).

Phase 5: Implementation

The Compass Strategy program was implemented over a three-year period. The core message of the media campaign evolved from the preliminary phases of the PPM. In addition to one core message, the researchers created five other messages based upon the predisposing and reinforcing factors and the Health Belief Model constructs related to seeking help. Researchers determined the channels of communication for the campaign by reviewing focus group responses and survey findings. Major and minor media were reviewed and analyzed based on the ability to accurately disseminate the core messages and to adequately reach adolescents and parents.

A website and information line (hotline) were developed to provide information relative to the core messages and to address enabling factors to foster early detection and seeking-help skills. Video modules and Navigation Program workshops were developed to deal with all predisposing, reinforcing, and enabling factors. Intervention strategies were based upon two theoretical frameworks: (1) the Transtheoretical Model/Stages of Change, and (2) Diffusion of Innovations. Researchers chose these frameworks because individuals are in different readiness stages regarding willingness to contemplate mental illness.

Prior to implementation of the program, researchers pretested all forms of minor and major media outlets using a representative sample of the target population. The website was pretested to ensure ease of navigation and functionality. Video modules were constructed after consulting local education departments who utilized this form of media marketing channel. Each form of minor and major media communication channel served a different purpose and each channel had a separate implementation and evaluation plan. The implementation plans were based on the Transtheoretical Model/Stages of Change. The different media forms were implemented in different waves and varied in intensity to ensure appropriate timing for a robust impact. Thus, multiple media forms were used concurrently to mimic commercial marketing practices.

Phases 6–8: Process, Impact, and Outcome Evaluations

The process evaluation determined whether the Compass Strategy was implemented according to the established objectives and whether it was operating efficiently. Researchers developed a 65-item questionnaire that was utilized for the process evaluation. The items on the measure were linked to the program objectives and goals established within the strategic plan. The process evaluation assessed the program objective of creating appropriate campaigns for adolescents, parents, teachers, and community leaders. For example, the researchers created a "pop-up" questionnaire for the website which asked website users questions regarding age, gender, postal code, and referral source. Researchers tracked the number of hits on the website and the number of calls to the information hotline. They determined as the intensity of the campaign increased, the usage of the website and the information hotline also increased.

The researchers utilized the telephone interviews to complete the impact evaluation. Researchers took a baseline measure of 600 adolescents in the intervention group and 600 adolescents in the comparison group. Logistic regression was used to identify any associations between the campaign-outcome variables: group (intervention, comparison) and time (preintervention, postintervention). Researchers only considered a

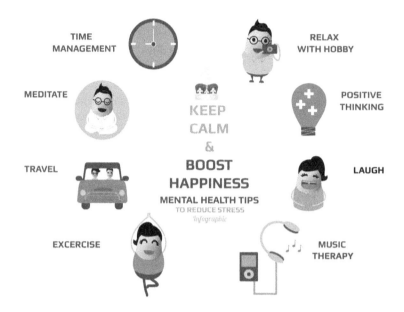

Figure 12.4.   Mental Health Tips.

© Shutterstock.com.

program impact if the group-by-time interaction was statistically significant. Statistical significance was found for the following outcome variables: (1) perceived suicide risk, (2) help seeking barriers, (3) media exposure, (4) correct prevalence exposure to media campaigns, and (5) self-identified depression. Additionally, there was a statistically significant change in the number of participants who were seeking help over time in the intervention group. For the outcome evaluation, researchers had planned to study changes in service utilization, length of untreated mental illness, and pathways to treatment; however, they were unable to collect the necessary data to complete the evaluation. Figure 12.4 illustrates different strategies to improve overall mental health.

Summary

Part V of this text book focuses on the application and evaluation of theory within the practice of health education. Theories are integral in advancing our understanding of the specific behavioral and environmental factors that influence health and health behaviors; however, theories must be properly integrated and applied to health promotion programs. This chapter provided an overview of one of the most widely utilized program planning models: the PRECEDE-PROCEED model (PPM). A brief history of the PPM was provided, as well as a detailed description of all eight phases. The phases of the PRECEDE-PROCEED Model include: (1) Social Assessment, (2) Epidemiological Assessment, (3) Educational and Ecological Assessment, (4) Administrative and Policy Assessment and Intervention Alignment, (5) Implementation, (6) Process Evaluation, (7) Impact Evaluation, and (8) Outcome Evaluation. The Compass Strategy program served as an applied example of the PPM relative to increasing mental health literacy among adolescents and the community in order to enhance awareness, early detection, and treatment of mental disorders.

References

Australian Health Ministers. (1998). Second National Mental Health Plan. Canberra, Australia: Mental Health Branch, Commonwealth Department of Health and Family Services.

Bartholomew, L. K., Parcel, G. S., Kok, G., & Gottlieb, N. H. (2001). *Intervention mapping: Designing theory- and evidence-based health promotion programs.* Mountain View, CA: Mayfield.

Bartholomew, L. K., Parcel, G. S., Kok, G., & Gottlieb, N. H. (2006). *Planning health promotion programs: An intervention mapping approach.* San Francisco: Jossey-Bass.

Gielen, A. C., McDonald, E. M., Gary, T. L., & Bone, L. R. (2008). Using the PRECEDE-PROCEED model to apply health behavior theories. In K. Glanz, B. K. Rimer, & K. Viswanath (Eds.), *Health behavior and health education: Theory, research, and practice* (4th ed., pp. 407–433). San Francisco: Jossey-Bass.

Gilmore, G. D. (2012). *Needs and capacity assessment strategies for health education and health promotion* (4th ed.). Burlington, MA: Jones & Bartlett Learning.

Green, L. W., & Kreuter, M. W. (2005). *Health promotion planning: An educational and ecological approach* (4th ed.). New York: McGraw-Hill.

Green, L. W., Kreuter, M. W., Deeds, S. G., & Partridge, K. B. (1980). *Health education planning: A diagnostic approach.* Mountain View, CA: Mayfield.

Institute of Medicine. (2003). *The future of the public's health in the 21st century.* Washington, DC: National Academy Press.

Institute of Medicine Committee on Health and Behavior. (2001). *The interplay of biological, behavioral, and societal influences, executive summary.* Washington, DC: National Academy Press.

Kretzmann, J. P., & McKnight, J. L. (1993). *Building communities from inside out: A path toward finding and mobilizing a community's assets.* Evanston, IL: Institute for Policy Research.

McKenzie, J. F., Neiger, B. L., & Smeltzer, J. L. (2005). *Planning, implementing & evaluating health promotion programs* (4th ed., pp. 15–52). San Francisco: Pearson Education.

Simons-Morton, B., McLeroy, K. R. & Wendel, M. L. (2012). *Behavior theory in health promotion practice and research.* Burlington, MA: Jones & Bartlett Learning.

Timmreck, T. C. (1997). *Health services cyclopedic dictionary* (3rd ed.). Boston: Jones & Bartlett.

Wright, A., McGorry, P. D., Harris, M. G., Jorm, A. F., & Pennell, K. (2006). Development and evaluation of a youth mental health community awareness campaign: The compass strategy. *BMC Public Health, 6* (215–13). doi:10.1186/1471-2458-6-215.

Chapter 12—Review Questions

1. Briefly describe the history of the PRECEDE-PROCEED model and how the current framework was created.

2. Identify and describe the planning phases of the PRECEDE-PROCEED model.

3. What are some common intervention strategies program planners would elect to utilize within a program?

4. Why is it necessary for the intervention strategies to match the selected behavioral and environmental determinants?

5. Compare and contrast predisposing, reinforcing, and enabling factors. Provide two examples for each.

6. What is a prioritization matrix? Why would program planners use this tool?

7. Define primary data and secondary data. When would a program planner collect these types of data?

8. In your own words, describe some of the activities that may take place during the Implementation phase of the PRECEDE-PROCEED model.

9. Describe the purpose of each of the three evaluation phases in the PRECEDE-PROCEED model.

10. The Compass Strategy program served as an applied example of the PRECEDE-PROCEED model. Research some local health promotion programs within your community and identify and describe one that may have utilized PRECEDE-PROCEED as a planning model.

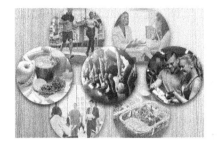

CHAPTER 13
The Health Education Process for Healthy Behavior Change and Needs Assessment

The health education process is at the core of behavior changes for successful health impacts and outcomes that improve health and the quality of life. The health education process includes needs assessment, program planning, program implementation, and program evaluation. The health education specialist has great responsibility in producing effective programs and interventions that result in responsible behavior change for improved health and quality of life. In fact, these components of the process represent four of the areas of responsibility for the health education specialists. Successful program development and intervention is dependent upon effective needs assessment, planning, implementation, and evaluation.

Needs assessment is the process by which the health education specialist identifies the issues, the needs, and problems that challenge our citizens and communities. The needs assessment identifies the target population most affected by the problems and their characteristics. The needs assessment also includes the identification of resources that individuals and populations can bring to meet their challenges.

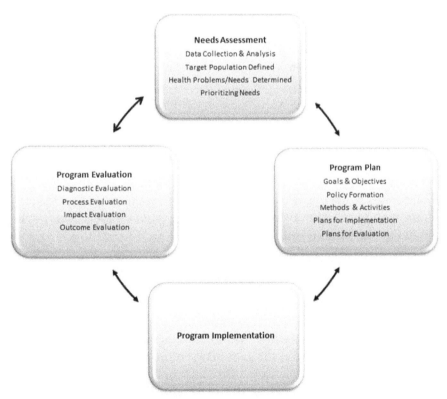

Figure 13.1. Health Education Process for Improved Quality of Life
© Kendall Hunt Publishing Company

Program planning is the process of determining the most effective ways to address the problems and needs of the target population who are most affected by the problems and who will receive the services to be offered; the nature of the services to be offered; and how resources should be applied.

The *implementation* process makes the plan reality through hiring and assigning trained staff; scheduling and actually offering the program services; marketing the program, and interacting with the consumers and target populations.

Evaluation is the process of monitoring program resources, services and the clients to determine program quality and effectiveness. Evaluation allows planned opportunities to answer questions about program effectiveness and about the continuance of program activities.

These components of the health education process are often presented separately, but when they are effectively administered, the boundaries are not so clearly distinguishable. Simons-Morton, Greene and Gottlieb (1995) described the interrelationships of planning, implementation and evaluation similar to biological processes: "A healthy program is like a healthy organism with the planning process as a central nervous system responding to the sensory feedback of evaluation and directing the muscles of implementation."

Breckon et al., (1998) suggested that the health education process requires planning for every aspect of the process for health education programming. The planning process involves planning with people, planning with data, planning for permanence, planning for priorities, planning for measurable outcomes in acceptable formats, and planning for evaluation. The following gives an overview of these planning concerns which are included in the process.

Plan with people. The people involved with the planning team must include representatives from the target population who are respected by the community, opinion leaders, and competent and trusted health professionals.

Plan the needs assessment process. The planners must determine the kinds of information and data that will be necessary to do effective program planning and how it will be collected, and by whom it will be collected and reported.

Plan with data. The data gathered through the needs assessment will be critical in directing the planning process. It is central to identifying health problems, issues, and resources.

Plan the program implementation. Planning is required in the effective selection and training of program staff, the marketing of the program, the recruitment of participants, the quality of services to the target population, the building of collaborations and partnerships, and in the administration of the program.

Plan the program evaluation. An effective plan for the program will provide for systematic and timely collection and analysis of information for successful program performance and decision-making.

Plan for dissemination of program progress, results and reports. Several individuals and groups must be involved and informed in the progress and outcomes of the program, such as the planners, their supervisors, administrators, community leaders, funding organizations, the target population, cooperating community agencies and organizations, etc.

Needs Assessment

The first important task of program planning is the *needs assessment.* The needs assessment allows for the examination of the health status of persons, specific groups, or the community, the identification of problems or issues, and the related factors. Perhaps the best definition for needs assessment is the process by which the health professional determines and measures the gaps between the population's health needs and the health care and health promotion services available to improve the population's health. Needs assessment is actually part of the evaluation and is also known as the diagnostic evaluation in program evaluation. This part of the planning process involves the collection of data that helps to identify individual, family and community resources, assets, and community stakeholders and leadership. The health education specialist and the planning committee must determine the purpose and scope of the needs assessment. What is to be gained by the assessment? Assessments can be informal and simple or formal and complex. This decision usually will be based on resources available and the expertise of the professional staff.

The needs assessment is that part of the planning process that serves to identify a population's most critical health issues and problems. The needs assessment is a planned effort to become acquainted with the population, their community setting, and the environment. The assessment presents the health education specialist with the opportunity to know the population's needs and issues, existing resources, the gaps between the needs and the resources, before recommending solutions and actions. The needs assessment includes both formal and informal data collection. It also includes the perceptions and values of the community leaders, groups, agencies, individuals and health organizations' staff about the health issues, problems, assets, barriers, and priorities for a given population. The data that is collected can include specific data and survey information to identify and verify the health status of a given population and the level of risk for that population. Without the needs assessment, there is no way to determine what services, programs, and policies are needed for which populations. While the needs assessment is used as the logical starting point of program planning, it is also an important method for monitoring change within the population being studied.

Who Is Involved in the Needs Assessment?

The practitioners of health education and health promotion focus on the goal of helping people (individuals, families, groups, and communities) choose patterns of behaviors which move them toward optimal health rather than toward disease. The goal includes helping these people to have the abilities to avoid many of the imbalances, diseases, and accidents of life. Therefore it is very important that the people who will receive the intervention and those who will be involved in the planning and implementation of the intervention work together in the overall planning process. The individuals who will be involved in the program must be involved *actively* in the planning—from conception through evaluation. The following individuals and groups should be considered as active participants in the process:

- Community members who will be clients/consumers
- Community leaders and stakeholders
- Health professionals serving the specific community
- Community elders
- Spiritual leaders
- Professionals officially responsible for the program plan

The health education specialist may actually select and recruit members of the above community groups and establish an advisory group for the project.

Health education specialists find community involvement very helpful and important in the health education process. Unfortunately, in many programs and services, there has been little, if any, community or tribal participation beyond the data collection. The results of not including representatives of the target population and the community throughout the process are that problems are poorly defined; the intervention misses the community context of the issues; the cultural context for the intervention is often missing; and the findings, conclusions, and assumptions are often incomplete, if not erroneous. Community involvement in the intervention usually means that problems such as trust issues and the lack of understanding among the target group to receive services, can be avoided. This growing role for community participation can also lead to the growing emphasis on self-determination in many communities, community empowerment, and the elimination of controversial and stigmatizing research and intervention outcomes that may produce negative stereotypes. Community members can help health education and health promotion professionals identify the differences between the values of the dominant culture and those of other cultures that can dictate the success for programs.

The relationships that planners and researchers have with the individuals, groups, and communities with whom they work must be firmly grounded in mutual respect, trust, and honesty. The quality of these relationships requires health education specialists to work with various populations from varied races, ethnicities, values, belief systems, spiritual and religious backgrounds, and genders. It is vital that health education specialists are culturally sensitive and culturally competent in the execution of all responsibilities and services. Cultural competence is central to developing trusting and respectful relationships. The health education specialist is expected to provide learning opportunities and experiences to help the population receiving services to also develop cultural competence so that they can better navigate the health care systems to receive appropriate and needed services. The Joint Committee on Terminology in Health Education and Health Promotion (2012, p. 16) defines cultural competence as "A developmental process defined as a set of values, principles, behaviors, attitudes, and policies that enable health professionals to work effectively across racial, ethnic and linguistically diverse populations."

Target Population

All of the information collected for each of the tasks listed below will contribute to identifying the target population and the issues that the planners will address. The target population is the group that is determined to be at risk for health problems or challenges based on the collected data. The target population is the population group that is being considered and will receive the benefits of the program being planned. It is the health of the target group that becomes the focus of the planned intervention.

Required Tasks for the Needs Assessment

The health professional must have a plan for the needs assessment that includes data collection from a variety of credible sources in order to accomplish the following:

1. Determination of the current health status of the target population.
2. Inventory of community assets and resources available to the community's populations.
3. Determination of the populations' use of existing health services.
4. Perceptions of the health providers regarding the elderly, disabled, maternal, child and youth health needs, since these are usually the most vulnerable population groups. However, other vulnerable and at-risk populations may be identified by the health providers.
5. Perceptions of the community regarding the elderly, disabled, maternal, child and youth health needs, since these are usually the most vulnerable population groups. However, other vulnerable and at-risk populations may be identified by the community.
6. Identification of the variables, factors and indicators from the health system, providers, individuals, families, community and environment that affect the population's health status and the health system.
7. Analysis of the collected data to define the health problem(s) or issue(s).
8. Establishment of priorities for addressing the health problem or issues of the defined target population.

Data Collection: Using the Professional Literature in the Health Education Process

The needs assessment reveals the current conditions, quality of life, and health status of the target population through data collection and analyses. The data collected must reflect the viewpoint of the health professionals and the viewpoint of the target population (perceived or actual needs). The sources of data for a needs assessment are varied and dependent upon the concerns of a given community and the planners.

The health education process requires much knowledge and experience from those responsible for program planning. The target populations and the communities will supply a great amount of credible qualitative and quantitative data that will be important to the planning efforts. However, one of the most important resources that professionals in health education and health promotion can readily access is the vast stores of literature available in print and electronic formats. Not only does this resource help the professional health educator in the planning process, but it also provides the health education specialist with an ever expanding source of information. This information is important to fulfilling the responsibilities of serving as a health education resource person and advocating for health and health education. There has been an explosion in the health literature that is available, because of the increasing demand to know more about health issues. Needless to say, all health education specialists would be wise to consult with and gain the assistance of a reference librarian (Cottrell et al., 2012). Fulfilling the areas of responsibility in health education requires accessing and using data. The sources of data used by the health education specialist for the needs assessment may be primary, secondary, or tertiary.

The primary sources of data are eyewitness accounts and studies with data collected personally by the planner that answers unique questions related to specific data needs. Primary data that one personally collects may be from conducted experiments, interviews, focus groups, surveys, questionnaires, or personal records that relate to the topic in question (McKenzie et al., 2013). Primary data has the advantage of directly addressing questions that health program planners want answered by the target population. However, primary data can be expensive given the time and financial resources that may be required in collecting, analyzing, and reporting the data. Primary research data or information is often published in peer reviewed or referred journals. Many of these journals are available in print or electronic formats. Peer reviewed journals are those which publish articles only after the manuscripts have been reviewed and accepted by panels of experts.

Secondary data are those data already collected and published by someone else and are available for your use. The advantage of using secondary data is that they already exist, so there is minimal time spent in data collection; and accessing secondary data is usually inexpensive. Secondary sources of data are usually published in journals or books. Journals may be peer-reviewed or refereed. Secondary data can also be found in governmental publications and in credible nongovernmental agencies and organizations. These agencies will usually provide formal publications of their data for use by professionals through free print or electronic access. Most colleges and universities serve as repositories for these data sources. Some sources for secondary data include:

- National, state, and local health status and vital statistics annual reports
- Epidemiological data
- County and city information from different organizations, hospitals, and health units
- Records of health and health care
- Health Risk Appraisals or Health Hazard Appraisals
- Historical accounts
- Peer-reviewed research findings and current literature
- Internet sources that are credible (May include websites of professional health organizations that are governmental or nongovernmental)

Tertiary sources of data are data collected from primary and secondary sources and refined to be included in handbooks, manuals, informational brochures serving the purposes of specific agencies or organization. This data would also include that which appears in encyclopedias, almanacs, dictionaries, fact books and other reference sources. Information from these sources is usually regarded as fact by the scientific community (Cottrell et al., 2012). Information that has no documentation to support its credibility and is replete with opinions intended for marketing a product is not tertiary data. These sources are classified as a fourth type of literature: popular press publications. These are usually magazine articles or editorials which are often biased. Information from the popular press must be scrutinized before confirming them as authentic, accurate or credible.

Because there is such a great need for data in the health education process, it is important that the planner knows how to conduct a literature search. It is fortunate that health education specialists have access to the internet and literature databases. Libraries in universities, colleges, and communities can provide access to databases. Databases can provide comprehensive listings of citations for journal articles, book chapters, books and access to abstracts of the literature. Most databases can identify sources by both author and subject or title. Some of the most common databases used by professionals in health education and health promotion are listed here.

PubMed or Medline is a database provided by the US National Library of Medicine.

Education Resource Information Center (ERIC) sponsored by the Institute of Education Sciences (IES), US Department of Education.

PsycINFO produced by the American Psychological Association.

Web of Science (Web of Knowledge) sponsored by Thomas Reuters.

EBSCO *host* provided by EBSCO Publishing.

Google Scholar provided by Google.

The following steps should help in a literature search.

Step 1 Identify the data need or topic that is to be searched. Search by subject or title or by author's last name. If the topic cannot be found, use other key words with similar meanings. Use a thesaurus if necessary.

Step 2 Search the topic or author in the database by the publication years of interest.

Step 3 From the results of your search, identify the possible data sources that meet the need or topic.

Step 4 Locate the literature sources in print or electronically.

Step 5 By reviewing the abstracts or the entire document, determine the quality and usefulness of the data sources or publications to the needs assessment process.

Step 6 Examine the references in the article. This may lead the planner to other data sources that may be useful.

Step 7 Keep a listing of all sources with full citations so that it can be easily transferred to the intervention plan's reference list or bibliography. The planner must always cite and reference all data used in the process.

Primary Data Collection Methods

Primary data collection is important because it can provide accurate population-specific data about problems, influences, and potential solutions to health issues. Collecting primary data through surveys, interviews, and focus group interviews can help the health education specialist establish important relationships with the community and its residents. Primary data collection methods are individual assessments and group assessments.

Individual assessments include surveys, the Delphi technique and interviewing. A survey is a structured method of gathering information directly from the individual by asking questions. Answers to questions may be obtained by mailed surveys that are returned by mail. Telephone surveys and face to face surveys are other options. When using survey methods, the health professional must be sure that the data collected is representative of the target population. The planner must address the questions of how the survey sample is chosen, and whether the survey instrument is valid and reliable. The valid survey instrument must measure what it is intended to measure. The reliable survey instrument must provide consistent results with subsequent use.

The Delphi technique is used when objective information is not available from other means. The Delphi technique generates "a consensus of opinion within a group through a series of questions. The process usually involves three to five rounds of mailed questionnaires in which the participants are asked to respond to general questions in the first round. From these responses more specific questions are asked with each successive round. This becomes a good technique to identify goals and establish priorities in a group or to clarify issues important to the group.

The interviewing method is unique and can encourage participation, but it is very dependent on the interviewer's skill in obtaining data from the interviewee. Establishing rapport and trust with the interviewee are key factors.

There are many trade-offs between cost of data collection and quality of the data obtained. The cost of data collection and summarization tends to increase as we move along the spectrum of mail surveys, telephone surveys, face-to-face surveys, interviews, and medical examinations. Butler (2001) notes the advantages and disadvantages of each. To choose a method of data collection, examine the advantages that may include: affordable cost, acceptable time frames, accuracy of data, honesty of answers, privacy and convenience of the respondent, likely rates of return (response or completion rates), degree to which complex vs. standardized questions can be asked, and scientific validity of the resulting data. In-person surveys and interviews may have the added advantages of building trust between the interviewer and interviewee and increasing morale in the community.

On one end of the continuum, mail surveys are relatively quick and inexpensive, and the individual's privacy can be protected, at least on the surveyor's end, so that answers may be more honest. However, the mailing list may be inaccurate, there is no ability to determine who answers the questions, rates of return may be low, and the returned surveys may be incomplete. In addition, questions need to be simple, and there is no opportunity to clarify them for the respondents. On the other end of the continuum, medical examinations are costly, but highly accurate and quantitative. Honoring the privacy of potential respondents and keeping participants' data confidential is very important, and laws about private health information such as the Health Insurance Portability and Accountability Act (HIPAA) may come into play. In every incidence of collecting data, participants must give their informed consent to participate in the data collection protocol.

Whereas standardized surveys and medical examinations may provide quantitative data about groups, key informant interviews allow for in-depth, nuanced, qualitative data which may provide insights into the context and dimensions of issues in the community. Interviewers must be highly trained, and the very richness of the data may make data analysis time-consuming and difficult. This method allows for considerable trust to be built between the interviewer and interviewee, but embarrassing or threatening questions might not be answered accurately.

In between mailed surveys and interviews are telephone and face-to-face surveys. Interviewers can help to assure survey completion, and questions can be somewhat more complex than in mailed surveys. However, key groups may not have telephones, or may not be willing to answer a telephone for this purpose, "interviewer bias" may occur if the interviewer changes the questions, or the subjects may change their answers so as to be more socially acceptable.

The group assessments include nominal group process, focus group interviews and forums. Nominal group process is a highly structured process that allows researchers or planners to qualify and quantify specific needs of a target population. The group consists of five to seven participants who have some understanding of the issues being considered. The members are asked to write their answers to a question without discussion. Each member then shares one response in a round-robin fashion until each response from every member has been heard by the group. Participants then vote to select and rank the number of items they think are most important related to the issue of concern.

Focus group interviews first began as a method in group therapy. It then evolved as a marketing technique that seeks to understand consumer behavior. Focus groups have been used successfully in a variety of settings. They are used in an exploratory manner to generate information about attitudes, opinions and hypotheses and to test new ideas. Focus groups are usually six to twelve members. The focus group is usually low cost, but the small group size makes it difficult to generalize findings to larger populations.

Community forum is less structured than other group assessments and can involve greater numbers of participants. Community forums are public meetings. They are useful for distributing information in a community, but can also generate initial feedback on topics presented to the community. The community forum allows all community members and groups to voice their opinions and concerns. The caution is to not let the forum degenerate into a gripe session.

Determining the Status of Existing Health Programs

Besides determining the health status of the target population, the status of health programs must also be determined. This also involves data collection methods similar to those already presented. Secondary data sources and primary data sources about the target population, the health care professionals and community leaders, can offer great insights and data to answer the following questions.

1. What are the programs and services available and accessible to the target population? Remember to examine all sources of services—public health organizations, community health organizations, volunteer organizations, religious organizations, etc.
2. What is the geographic proximity of the services to the population?
3. Are the programs and services utilized by the target population, and to what extent?
4. Are the programs and services meeting their organizational stated goals and objectives?
5. What is the actual cost of the service to the target population as consumers and to the taxpayer?
6. Are the services culturally appropriate and competent for the population(s) being served?
7. Are the needs of the target population being met? If not, why?
8. Are there available programs and services leading to positive changes in the quality of life for the target population?
9. Are there gaps in the services offered?
10. To what extent are services coordinated with other health and health-related services?

Analyzing the Data

Once the required data are collected, the health education specialist and the planning team must analyze the data to identify and prioritize problems and needs of the target population and those who will serve them. Due to limited funding and resources, setting priorities among the identified needs is warranted, since there are usually not enough resources to address all needs. After collecting the data, the health professional must analyze all of the data. The analysis of the data may be formal or informal. The formal analysis usually involves statistical analysis. The informal analysis which is used most often is commonly known as **eyeballing the data** (Windsor et al., 1984). Eyeballing the data simply means looking at the data for differences between what exists and what ought to be. Again, the health education specialist must review and analyze the data according to the original plan of the needs assessment, answering the following questions.

- How can the target population be best described and defined?
- What is the current health status of the target population?
- What are the resources available to the community and target populations?
- How are the populations using the existing health services?
- What are the perceptions of the health providers regarding maternal, child and youth health needs?
- What are the perceptions of the community and the target populations regarding maternal, child, and youth health needs?
- Which variables, factors, indicators or precursors from the health system, providers, individuals, families, community and environment are identified as affecting the population's health status and the health system?
- Finally, define and describe the problems that the needs assessment has revealed to the planners.

Data analysis can be straightforward when there is agreement across all the data for a given issue. However, this may not be the case in situations in which the data for morbidity does not support the mortality data; or where the target population's perceptions of key health issues do not correspond with the data from the health care providers in the same community.

McKenzie et al., (2013), suggest that using the first few phases of the PRECEDE PROCEED Model provides guidance in the problem analysis by answering the following questions:

1. Starting with Phase 1, what is the quality of life for the target population? Why did this group become the priority and focus of the needs assessment?
2. What are the actual and perceived social circumstances shared by those in the target population?
3. What are the social indicators in the target population that reflect these conditions (e.g., crime, absenteeism, school performance, poverty, unemployment, discrimination)? Do the statistical data support these findings?
4. Can the social conditions be linked to determinants of health addressed by health promotion?
5. Can these social conditions be linked to health problems? What are the health problems? How does the data support the linkage?
6. Which health problem(s) is most important for change and receives top priority for health education and health promotion efforts?

Problem Diagnosis

The sixth question is essential in identifying a prioritized list of problems and needs that the program plan will address. The planner must now complete the problem diagnosis. In examining the list of problems, the planner must have a clear understanding of which problems will set the direction and priorities for programs or interventions. This means that the planners must be able to identify the variables, factors, indicators and/ or precursors that relate to or cause the identified problem and impact health status. Given the identified problem, what are the social and health consequences of the health problem? The planner addresses the core variables of the identified problem through problem diagnosis. A systematic diagnosis of a health problem or need has four distinct stages: per-ception, verification, setting priorities, and analysis (Peoples-Sheps MD, et al., 1996).

Perception

The perception of the problem is usually defined as the gap that exists between what is (the real) and what should be (the ideal). The perception of health problems must be addressed from the health education specialists' viewpoints and from the target populations' viewpoints. Ideally, if there is good communication among these groups and a strong working relationship, then there will not be great differences between the perceptions of needs for these groups. Therefore it is important to involve the target population throughout all phases of program development. The task of collecting data to determine this has been presented earlier. The need to collect data about suspected problems is to establish that the problem is not just someone's opinion or personal concern, but it is rooted in actual data. Indicators of health status and the ideal levels or the recommended levels for those indicators are required in diagnosing health problems and needs of the target population. The incidences of diseases or other health statistics are usually used as measures of health conditions. In other situations a variable or a risk factor may be highly predictive of a health problem, and will be measured in place of measuring the actual health problem or need. An example of this would be the measurement of incomplete DPT immunization status ". . . may be considered a surrogate indicator for a health problem, because a child who does not receive the full DPT series is at higher risk for diphtheria, pertussis, and tetanus than a child who receives the full immunization series" (Peoples-Sheps MD, et al., 1996). There are also situations when one risk factor contributes to several health conditions (e.g., smoking). Then using the risk factor as the focus for assessing multiple health status indicators may be efficient and productive.

In discussing problem perception, a word of caution is needed. It is most important not to define health problems as a service delivery deficiency. If this occurs, the planners are likely to focus on the lack of services or programs rather than a health problem. For an example, a health professional may observe that many of the high-risk prenatal clients bring their pre-school children to the clinic when they come for prenatal health care. Instead of the health care planners focusing on the health status of the prenatal clients and their real needs, they begin to plan child care or nursery services for the clients. While these services may be helpful, there is no evidence that the lack of child care service is a health problem for the target population. Kiritz (1980) refers to defining missing services as a problem as circular reasoning. The danger of this circular reasoning is that once the missing services are provided and the population part-icipates in the services, the health care providers may declare that the problem is solved. However, the real problem has not been defined, because there is inadequate needs assessment. The needs for the pregnant women in this example are unmet. The focus of the development of health education and health promotion programs is to be responsive to the populations' health problems or unmet health needs, and not to spurious observations that have little to do with the real health needs of the population.

The health problem or unmet need has been defined as the difference between *what is* and *what should be*. The health education specialist's job is to determine the nature of the identified problem. When the true nature and context of the problem is determined, there may be many ways to intervene and many resources to be used. So problem diagnosis is essential to understand the problem, its characteristics, dynamics, its magnitude and severity, and its cause(s) or precursors. It is only when this diagnostic process is complete that the planners get clearer insights into how to effectively and efficiently address the defined problem(s).

Problem Verification

The verification process examines several aspects of the problems observed in the needs assessment to determine if the findings are really problems. The health education specialist must determine the extent of the identified problem(s), its duration, its expected future course and costs, and its variation across the community's population groups and geographic areas. Using the responses to the following questions, the health education specialist can verify that the identified problems are really problems for the target population:

1. What do you already know about the problem?
2. What information about the problem is missing?
3. Gather information on the problem—its causes and precursors, its characteristics, its incidence, its prevalence.
4. How many people are affected? What percentage of the total population do they represent?
5. How long has the problem been observed at the current level?
6. In what ways has the problem changed over time?
7. Clarify the definition(s) of the problem(s).

Setting Priorities

Public health and community health agencies are always faced with the dilemma of solving many health problems with limited resources: human, financial, or other resources. It becomes necessary to set priorities among problems and decide how to allocate limited resources to solving the problems. What must be the criteria for setting priorities for health problems? The criteria are not always straightforward because both the criteria and the problems may be controversial. It is not as simple as choosing problems that have serious consequences over those that have less serious consequences. Both types of problems may have controversial aspects. So in determining the criteria for prioritizing problems, it is important to have as much input from as many stakeholders as possible. The group of stakeholders should include representatives from the target population, state and local agencies, community organizations and businesses. It is essential that planners plan for equal and balanced input from all participants.

The following questions can indicate suggested criteria by which the program planner(s) may decide to set priorities among identified problems

1. Through the verification process, is the problem important? What is the pressing need?
2. Is it feasible to solve the problem? Are there adequate resources available to address the problem?
3. Are you the best people to solve the problem? Are others best suited to solve the problem? Who are they?
4. Have you weighed the positive and negative impacts of solving and not solving the problem?
5. Can the problem be solved in a reasonable time frame? Explain.

Problem Analysis

After completing the above process for identifying and prioritizing the health problems, the health education specialist and the planning committee should be ready to move forward to the final stage of problem analysis and developing a problem statement. According to Witkin and Altschuld (2000), there are many ways to analyze each problem. However, it is generally recommended that the planner consider a broad range of precursors and consequences that represent all domains of the problem for the target population and health care providers. It would be helpful to diagram the problem and these domains to help conceptualize the problem and its various characteristics. Such a diagram could be helpful in the development of the program plan.

Peoples-Sheps et al., (1996) suggests the use of a problem diagram. The problem diagram presented in Figure 13.2 has four components: the problem, the precursors to the problem, the consequences of the problem, and linkages. There is no real right or wrong way to illustrate these diagrams. The goal is to find the best way to demonstrate the precursors and consequences of a problem. In this diagram the problem appears in the middle of the diagram. The precursors are in the upper portion of the diagram and the consequences appear in the lower portion of the diagram. In both portions the precursors and the consequences are listed in the order of direct to secondary and to tertiary factors related to the problem. The arrows indicate the known and/ or the hypothesized linkages. The precursors are factors associated with the problem. Some are directly linked and others are indirectly linked. The problem diagram presented here is for the hypothetical problem of low birthweight in Mercer County, AnyState, USA.

In the problem diagram, the precursors are the factors that influence, are strongly related to, and/or may be a cause of the problem of low birthweight. The consequences that appear in the diagram are the direct or indirect effects of the problem on the individual, family, and society. The health education specialist has learned about the precursors and consequences through the data collected in the needs assessment and through the professional literature and research generated about low birthweight.

It is important to note that the consequences of one cycle of the problem may become precursors of the next as indicated by the arrow connecting poverty in the consequences to the poverty in the precursor section. At the end of such a problem analysis, the health professional and others working as part of the planning team should have a clear conceptualization of the problem and all of the factors related to it.

The epidemiological and relative risk literature will help with the identification of the linkages. Relative risk is measured by an odds ratio, and is an indicator of the strength of the association between a risk factor and a health problem. This measurement is the ratio of the incidence of the problem in the population of people with the risk factor to the incidence in the population without the risk factor. Relative risk indicators can be used to identify risk factors for the problem diagram and to help determine the potential impact of

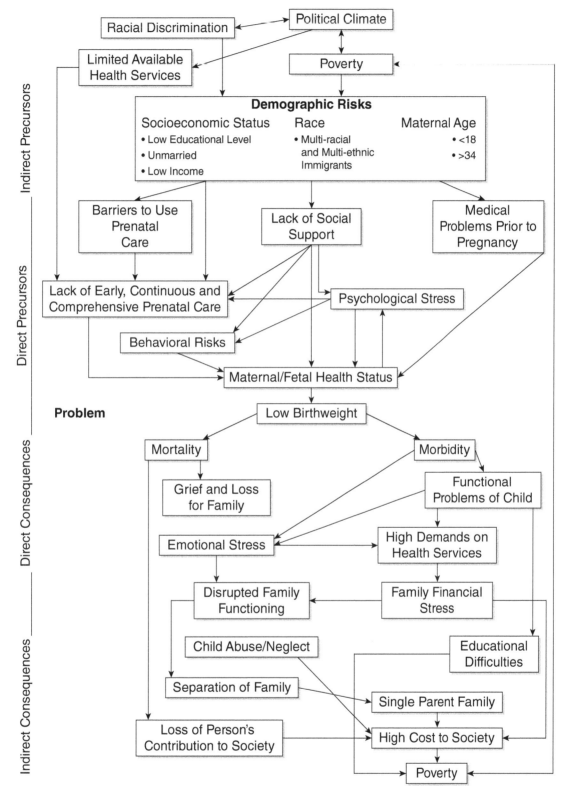

Figure 13.2.   Problem diagram of low birthweight in Mercer County, Any State, USA

intervening at a specific precursor. One example of this would be the comparative impacts of maternal smoking and maternal alcohol consumption. If maternal smoking has a higher relative risk for low birthweight than maternal alcohol consumption, then an intervention that is directed towards smoking cessation for pregnant women would potentially have more of an impact on low birthweight than an intervention that focuses on reducing alcohol consumption.

The Problem Statement

The health education specialist and the planning committee have completed the problem analysis. Now it is time to write the problem statement. The problem statement may be about two paragraphs in length and will include the following information:

- The defined condition, situation, or issue.
- Explain why the condition is sufficiently prevalent to be considered a problem?
- Which subgroups in the population are disproportionately affected by the problem? How are they affected?
- What is known about the relationships among precursors, consequences and the problem?
- Which of the direct and indirect precursors are more prevalent in the studied community compared to other communities?
- What are the precursors that the program will address to solve the problem?
- Which of the consequences will be relieved or eliminated as a result of reducing or eliminating the problem?
- Describe the target population who will be the focus of the program or intervention.

Reporting the Results of the Needs Assessment

The planners responsible for the needs assessment have completed the essential and initial tasks of the needs assessment. As a result of the needs assessment, the health problem(s) and/or issues have been identified and clearly defined. The results of the needs assessment should be shared with all members of the planning team, their administrators, the target population and its official representatives, other community stakeholders, as a formal report.

The health professional responsible for program development has completed the essential and initial tasks of the needs assessment of data collection and analysis. As a result of this process, the health problem(s) and/or issues have been identified. Next the planner must examine and clearly diagnose the problem(s), set priorities, develop a problem statement, develop the hypothesis for the recommended intervention, and develop realistic goals and objectives for the program.

References

Agency for Healthcare Research and Quality. 1995. *The Future of Children: Low Birthweight.* AHRQ Publication No. 00-P010. Rockville, MD. http://ahrq.gov/clinic/lobrhigh.htm.

Breckon, J., J. R. Harvey, and R. B. Lancaster. 1998. *Community Health Education: Settings, roles, and skills for the 21st Century.* Gaithersburg, MD: Aspen Publishers, Inc.

Butler, J. T. 2001. *Principles of Health Education and Health Promotion* (3rd ed.). Belmont, CA: Wadsworth/ Thomas Learning.

Coreil, J., C. A. Bryant, and J. N. Henderson. 2001. *Social and Behavioral Foundations of Public Health.* Thousand Oaks, CA: Sage.

Cottrell, R. R., J. T. Girvan, and J. F. McKenzie. 2012. *Principles and Foundations of Health Promotion and Education.* Boston: Benjamin Cummings.

Doyle, E., and S. Ward. 2005. *The Process of Community Health Education and Promotion.* Long Grove, IL: Waveland Press, Inc.

Estes, G., and D. Zitow. 1980. *Heritage Consistency as a Consideration in Counseling Native Americans.* Paper read at the National Indian Education Association Convention, Dallas, TX.

Giger, J. N., and R. E. Davidhizar. 1995. *Transcultural Nursing Assessment and Intervention*, 2nd ed. St. Louis: Mosby-Year Book.

Joint Committee on Health Education and Promotion Terminology. (2012). Report of the 2011 Joint Committee on Health Education and Promotion Terminology. *American Journal of Health Education, 43* (2).

Kiritz, N. J. 1980. *Program Planning and proposal writing.* Los Angeles: The Grantsmanship Center.

McKenzie, J. F., B. L. Neiger, and R. Thackeray. 2013. *Planning, Implementing, and Evaluating Health Promotion Programs: A Primer.* Boston: Pearson Education.

Peoples-Sheps MD, A. Farel, and M. M. Rogers. 1996. *Assessment of Health Status Problems.* Washington, DC: Maternal and Child Health Bureau.

Simons-Morton, B. G., W. H. Greene, and N. H. Gottlieb. 1995. *Introduction to Health Education and Health Promotion.* Prospect Heights, IL: Waveland.

Specter, R. 2009. *Cultural Diversity in Health and Illness.* Upper Saddle River, NJ: Pearson/Prentice Hall.

Windsor, R., T. Baranowski, N. Clark, and G. Cutter. 1984. *Evaluation of Health Promotion and Education Programs.* Palo Alto, CA: Mayfield.

Witkin, R., and J. Altschuld. 2000. Planning and Conducting Needs Assessments. Thousand Oaks, CA, Sage. Yomiuri (2000).

Application Opportunity

1. Identify credible sources of health data nationally, in your home state, and in your local community (county, district, or city). List these sources below.

2. Use these sources to determine the ten (10) leading causes of mortality nationally, in your home state and in your local community. Are the 10 leading causes of mortality the same for national, state, and local statistics?

1. Examine the number 1 cause of mortality in your local community and determine what segment of the population is carrying the greatest disease burden for that cause of mortality. Describe what you see in the data by race/ethnic groups, sex, and age.

2. Research the health problem that you identified in item 1. List the risk factors or precursors and consequences for the health problem.

3. Illustrate your findings in a problem map. Attach the problem map to and submit the map with this Application Opportunity.

4 Can the problem be addressed by health education? Why or why not?

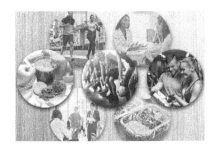

CHAPTER 14
Health Education Process: Developing the Program Plan

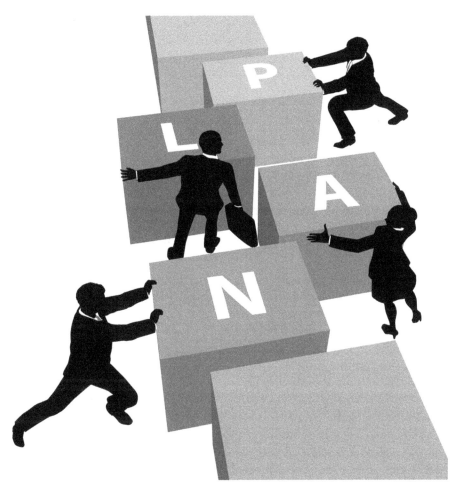

© Michael D. Brown, 2013, Used under license from Shutterstock, Inc.

Program planning is a complex process by which an intervention or program is designed to help meet the needs of a specific group of people, target population, or priority population. The health education specialist and the planning team will develop the hypothesis, goals, objectives, strategies in designing a program to meet the identified needs of the population that are identified in the needs assessment. The needs assessment produces a problem statement that is instrumental in developing a program plan. The contents of the problem statement are presented in the previous chapter. From the problem statement and other assessment findings the health education specialist should be able to produce a relevant and culturally appropriate program for the target population. See the example of a problem statement generated from the problem diagram presented in the previous chapter.

An Example of a Problem Statement for Low Birthweight Births in Mercer County

In Mercer County there is growing concern among its residents and health care providers about the increase in teen pregnancies over the past five years. A variety of health and social agencies are now addressing the goal of reducing teenage pregnancy with programs for both male and female adolescents. Along with this increase in teenage pregnancies, there is an increase in the births of low birthweight (LBW) babies. In 2008, the low birth weight rate for all women was 5.6% which was below the state low birthweight percentage of 6.8% in 2008. The goal for the state for low birthweight births was 5% by 2010, based on the Healthy People 2010 targets. However, by 2010, the LBW babies increased to 7.3% for the state and 9.7% for Mercer County. In 2012 the LBW percentage rose to 10.5% in Mercer County. While this problem is seen across racial and income groups, there are populations experiencing very high percentages of low birthweight births. Those who experience the highest percentages of LBW are adolescents 17 years old and under, members of newly arrived immigrant populations in urban areas of the county who are unmarried.

While teenage pregnancies are of great concern to the health care and social services professionals and the communities in Mercer County, LBW is of greater concern. Low birthweight babies are born weighing less than five pounds, eight ounces. Some low birthweight babies are healthy, even though they are small. But being low birthweight can cause serious health problems for some babies. There are two main reasons why a baby may be born with low birthweight: (1) premature births (babies born before 37 weeks of pregnancy; and Fetal growth restriction (small for gestational age). In the U. S. approximately seven of ten low-birthweight babies are premature. The earlier a baby is born, the lower the birthweight may be. About one in eight babies in the United States is born prematurely. Fetal growth restriction, the second reason for LBW births, results when the baby does not gain appropriate weight during the complete pregnancy.

The primary precursors for LBW births are lack of early, continuous and comprehensive care, psychological stress, behavioral risks (poor eating behaviors, poor nutrition, lack of personal hygiene, smoking) all of which impact on both the maternal and the fetal health status. The primary consequences of LBW are greater risks for infant mortality and morbidity that increase the emotional and economic stress for the mother, her family, and the infant. The consequences of LBW morbidity can continue and grow throughout childhood and adulthood.

The needs assessment reveals that the population experiencing the greatest percentage of LBW is a diverse population of recently arrived immigrants who are originally from eastern Europe, eastern Africa and Central America. Many of the population do not speak English. They do not know the health care system and especially do not seek prenatal care. The community is very low income with low literacy rates. Many cannot afford the costs of prenatal care so they do not seek it for pregnancy. Among those receiving care in the health clinics, there is adherence to traditional cultural practices that may be harmful to a developing fetus. For those teenagers who are pregnant and unmarried, shame may keep them from seeking care.

The Health Education and Health Promotion Committee for Healthy Pregnancies proposes a program to reduce low birthweight births in the city of Crawford in Mercer County. Such a program that will offer services to all pregnant women in Crawford will especially target pregnant adolescent and pregnant immigrant women, offering early prenatal care, education and support throughout their pregnancies and the first year of their babies' lives.

There are several good theories, models and frameworks that are useful in designing health education and health promotion programs. Some of these were presented in chapter six. There is no perfect model or framework that will accurately cover or predict all facets and outcomes of the program plan. However, every program design will include some specific components: the problem statement, the mission statement, the hypothesis, program goal(s), program objectives, program intervention methods, activities, an implementation plan and an evaluation plan.

Planning with People

The reader is reminded that the process of planning a health education program requires the contributions of the health education specialist as the planner, the target population, and other stakeholders in all aspects of the proposed program. The complexity of the planning process demands an organized and team approach to the process. This collaborative effort must allow representation and input from all who are involved in the decision-making. This will most often mean that the people and settings will be culturally diverse. Effective and collaborative work requires mutual respect for the diverse contributions and views of each member of the planning team and all of the stakeholders. The work of the planning group should result in the consensus of the group supporting a relevant program plan that truly meets the needs of all who are concerned.

Planning Assumptions

As the planning team designs a program to solve the health problem(s), it must consider the following assumptions that are characteristic of good planning. The overall assumption is that things do change in any environment.

- Factors in the external environment could affect the demand for the program. The planners must identify changing demographics in the target population and the community, new mandates, political changes, changes in services and resources that can affect the program plan and address them accordingly.
- Fiscal factors may change. Changes such as increased fees and funding cuts that may affect the program must be considered in the design of the program plan.
- There are consequences of all actions.

Planners must be able to predict the consequences of such changes. Examples of such planning assumptions are:

The number of monolingual Spanish speaking families in the service area of the Rural Health Project is expected to increase by 30% over the next three years. Therefore culturally competent Spanish speaking administrative and health care staff must be hired to serve the population.

The agency providing the educational materials used by the Rural Health Project will no longer produce the high quality promotional and health education brochures after this year because of funding cuts. Therefore the program must consider new suppliers of educational and promotional materials and the costs of such materials.

In these examples, the health education specialist would design the program's goals, objectives, methods, implementation, evaluation, and budgets to realistically consider the impact of these expected changes. The specifics of the assumptions are derived from the needs assessment.

The Hypothesis

As the health education specialist progresses through the needs assessment and problem analysis phases, it is clear that solving problems can be complicated. Before beginning any specific actions to address the defined problem(s), it is expected that the health education specialist first receive approval regarding the identified need and a mandate to proceed with the program design. The next step in designing the health program is formulating a hypothesis. Health issues and problems are complex and are often multifaceted, offering multiple opportunities and pathways to address a given problem. The health professional chooses a specific programmatic response to a health need based on (1) the logical determination of why the problem exists; (2) the understanding and application of the evidence-based literature; and (3) the application of appropriate theories, models, and/or frameworks in addressing changing health behaviors. The formulation of the hypothesis will link the problem analysis results to the proposed goals and objectives. "The hypothesis assures that there will be internal consistency among the program's components, and that the program can be evaluated" (Hanson, 1997, p. 7).

In the previous section, a sample health problem was presented for low birthweight births increasing in Mercer County. There are several precursors that are associated with the increase in the percentage of low birthweight babies being born in Mercer County (See the problem diagram on page 130 and the problem statement on page 138). The term precursor can also mean risk factor. The most direct precursors are maternal and fetal health status, behavioral risks, psychological stress, and the lack of early, continuous and comprehensive prenatal care. The behavioral risks include poor dietary pattern to support pregnancy, substance abuse, poor hygiene, risky sexual behavior during pregnancy and some cultural practices that may affect the pregnancy (pica consumption). At the secondary precursor level, the precursors are barriers to the use of prenatal care, the lack of social support, and medical problems prior to pregnancy. The primary and secondary precursors are generally impacted by availability of health services, poverty, discrimination, and the political climate controls the funds for available health services, but also has some relationship to the racial discrimination and poverty seen in Mercer County. The health education specialist examines these precursors or risk factors and links based on the most recent literature and the needs assessment data, and then determines which factors will be addressed by the program. The planners will want to choose those precursors or risk factors that will give the most powerful response and resolution to the problem.

In order to make the best choice of the precursors to address, the health education specialist ranks the factors by level of importance to the problem and changeability. The level of importance is how strongly the factor contributes to the problem: low, moderate, high. The changeability is the planner's determination of how likely the precursors and thus the problem, can be affected through intervention, given the available resources, political climate, individual and community responsiveness, etc. The program should be designed to address the most important and changeable factors that impact the problem the most for the target population.

Problem's Precursor/Risk Factor Analysis for Program Hypothesis

The following table has been constructed to help determine the level of importance and changeability of precursors or risk factors for the defined problem. The determination must be based on funding and other resources available to the planner as mandated by the employer or the agency's administration. The funding, the needs assessment results, and the most current analysis of the literature related to the problem and the target population are used in the determination of which problem precursors will be the focus of the program.

Problem: Increased LBW births among teen mothers ≤17 in Mercer County, Any State, USA.

The results of the precursor/risk factor analysis may have different responses to the importance and the likelihood of change from different health education specialists, based on their given target populations and the circumstances and resources of their communities and agencies.

Given the results of the analysis in Table 14.1, the precursors that are scored "high" as the most important to the problem and can most likely be changed through program interventions are:

- Behavioral risks (poor dietary pattern to support pregnancy, substance abuse, poor hygiene, risky sexual behavior during pregnancy and some cultural practices)
- Psychological stress
- Lack of early, continuous, and comprehensive prenatal care
- Barriers to the woman's use of prenatal care
- Lack of social support

The other factors are definitely important in reducing low birthweight births in Mercer County, but within the respective agency, the health education specialist may not have the means to make the greatest impact on the problem through these precursors. Through collaboration with other community agencies, stakeholders and resources the health education specialists may indeed be able to change these factors. For the purpose of this example for reducing low birthweight births, the focus will be on those precursors that scored high for both importance and changeability. The hypothesis will state what will happen to the health problem, if through effective and relevant programming the precursors can be reduced or eliminated. The hypothesis will also identify the consequences of such actions. The consequences will very likely be positive impacts and outcomes for the target population and the community. So based on the example's analysis, the hypothesis might be expressed as follows:

- If pregnant women are recruited for participation in the prenatal health program;
- If pregnant women with high risk behaviors improve their health status by adopting health behaviors for healthy pregnancies and babies by adopting recommended prenatal diet and nutrition and physical activity, as well as eliminating substance use and abuse and risky sexual relationships;

Table 14.1.   Precursor/Risk Factor Analysis for Program Planning

Precursors or Risk Factors Contributing to the Problem	Level of Importance (low, moderate, high)	Level of Changeability (low, moderate, high)
Maternal health status during pregnancy	High	Moderate
Fetal health status	High	Moderate
Behavioral risks (poor dietary pattern to support pregnancy, substance abuse, poor hygiene, risky sexual behavior during pregnancy and some cultural practices)	High	High
Psychological stress	High	High
Lack of early, continuous and comprehensive prenatal care	High	High
Barriers to woman's use of prenatal care (financial, language, transportation, cultural barriers)	High	High
Lack of social support	High	High
Medical problems before pregnancy	High	Moderate
Political climate	High	Moderate
Poverty	High	Low
Racial discrimination	High	High
Limited available health services (general health services for the general population)	High	Low

- If pregnant women adopt skills to reduce psychological stress during pregnancy;
- If pregnant women participate in early, continuous and comprehensive prenatal care that is available for all pregnant women in Mercer County;
- If pregnant women in Mercer County can identify resources that enable them to overcome barriers to using prenatal care (financial, language, transportation, cultural barriers);
- If pregnant women utilize social support resources in Mercer County;

Then, the percentage of low birthweight births in Mercer County will decline to 5% by December 30, 2020 with the following consequences:

- The barriers to women of all socioeconomic circumstances needing prenatal care will be reduced;
- There will be reduced infant mortality and morbidity rates in Mercer County among women receiving early, continuous and comprehensive health care;
- There will be improvement in the postnatal health status of the mothers and their children who received early and continuous prenatal care

The program hypothesis states the precursors that will be addressed or targeted in the program design in order to have the greatest impact on reducing the problem. The hypothesis also states the consequences or expected results of the program for the target population and the community. The hypothesis becomes the guide for developing the program plan and its components. It is important to note that in most of the precursors in our example health education will be appropriate, but it is also necessary to collaborate with other medical and social services to realize the decline in low birthweight births for Mercer county.

The Mission Statement

Most program plans begin with an overview or short narrative that describes the general purpose or direction of the proposed program. This narrative is usually referred to as a mission statement, program overview, program aim or statement of purpose. It gives the intent of the program and an indication of the philosophical perspective of the planning group that influences the goal(s), the objectives, the content and methods of the program. The health education specialist will be able to use the developed hypothesis in writing the mission statement, because the hypothesis does outline what the purpose or mission of the program will be.

Examples of mission statements

- The mission of the Women's HIV Prevention Program is to provide a range of services that will reduce the HIV infection rate among women of child-bearing age. It is expected that this program will result in the reduction of morbidity and mortality among women and children who are at risk, by preventing HIV infection.
- The Radiologic Services of Crawford City recognizes the importance of establishing and promoting healthy lifestyles among our employees. Healthy employees are productive and happy employees and citizens of this great city. This worksite health program will encourage employees at Radiologic Services to adopt healthy eating and physical activity behaviors to improve and maintain good health.
- Children are our most important resource in Mercer County. They must be cherished and protected from birth throughout life. The Mercer County Health Department understands that early, continuous and comprehensive prenatal care is a major investment in the lives of our citizens. This program, Upward Bound will provide the best start for our children through medical care and health education during pregnancy and into infancy.

Goals

Some health professionals use the terms **goals** and **objectives** as though they were the same, they are not the same. Goals are future events or outcomes toward which a given program or intervention is directed. Objectives are the steps that will be taken to reach or achieve the goal. Goals provide the destination, while objectives give us precise measurable directives to reach the destination.

Goals are general and broad statements of what will be achieved. Goals form the foundation for the program planning process. They must be clear and concise, and deal realistically with the problems and solutions of the target population (Butler, 2001). Goals are usually long-term, taking longer to complete than an objective. The goal(s) should be agreed upon by the planning group that is representative of all stakeholders.

Goals may or may not be written as complete sentences. Goals are often written in the infinitive verb form. Goals are usually not measurable by exact methods. There is no set number of goals that have to be stated in a program. Some programs will have only one goal while others will have several stated goals. In examining the developed hypothesis on reducing low birthweight births we have "if" and "then" statements. The "if" statements are the changes in the precursors or risk factors that will lead to the "then" statement. The "then" statement in the hypothesis becomes the program's goal.

Below are different ways the goal may be written.

The percentage of low birthweight births in Mercer County will decline

To reduce low birthweight births in Mercer County

To increase the number of full-term babies born at optimal birthweights

The goal statement usually includes:

1. Who or what will be affected?
2. What will change as a result of the program?

Other examples of goals.
- All cases of juvenile violence in Pico County schools will be eliminated
- To increase the consumption of fruits and vegetables among adult women in Barrett, USA.
- To reduce the incidence of HIV infection among women of child-bearing age

Objectives

As stated earlier, objectives are very specific and measurable steps that will lead to achieving goals. Objectives are smaller actions or steps that must be completed on the way to fulfilling or reaching a goal. Therefore they are crucial to any program plan, and much care must go into developing them and writing them.

Objectives provide the health education specialist and other professionals with a clearer direction for achieving the change, impact, or outcome that will be accomplished in the program. Objectives make the selection of program strategies, methods and activities easier to choose. The selection of clear achievable and measurable objectives will also make program evaluation possible. Objectives should be written to address the most important and changeable factors. In the hypothesis for the birthweight example, the 'If' statements that deal with the precursors or risk factors become the basis for objectives for the program's goal, if they are written in measurable terms. As the planners develop the objectives they must be sure that they also write objectives that can be measured in the evaluation process.

An example of a specific measurable objective in a program with the goal of reducing juvenile violence may have the following objective:

> By the end of the academic year, 60% of students actively enrolled and participating in the program will demonstrate the basic skills for defusing potentially violent encounters.

The example illustrates the important elements that must be present in well-written objectives. Well-written objectives provide the planners with the means to not only select effective strategies and methods, but also the means for an effective evaluation process. McKenzie et al., (2013, p. 143) provide the planners with these elements of the well-written objectives.

- The outcome to be achieved. (What will change?)
- The condition under which the outcome will be observed. (When will the change occur?)
- The criterion for deciding whether the outcome has been achieved. (How much change is proposed?)
- The priority population or the target population. (Who will change?)

The Outcome

The outcome is the first element and defines the status, action, behavior, or some other factor that will change as a result of the program. The outcome is usually the verb of the statement. So in the example, the outcome is reflected in the verb "demonstrate." The participants in this program will be expected to demonstrate very specific behaviors and skills: the basic skills for defusing potentially violent encounters. The demonstrated new knowledge and skills are assumed to lead to behavior that reduces violence in the schools. The verb "demonstrate" can be documented, so that the objective can be measured and evaluated. During the academic year how many students actually could "demonstrate" skills in defusing violent situations?

Listing of verbs related to cognitive, affective, and psychomotor domains can be helpful to the planner in writing objectives. The reader was introduced to the *The Bloom's Taxonomy of Educational Objectives* (Bloom, 1956), in Chapter 6. It has been instructive for educators for many years in finding appropriate verbs for specific and measurable objectives. Table 14.2 list a few verbs that can be used in objectives about changes in knowledge (cognitive domain), feelings and attitudes (affective domain), and skills and behaviors (psychomotor domain) that can be used for the outcome element in well-written objectives. These are verbs that relate to something that is measurable and observable.

Some verbs are not appropriate choices for outcomes because they cannot be measured nor observed. These would be verbs such as *know, appreciate,* and *understand,* which imply outcomes that cannot be measured, observed nor evaluated. So an example of a poor objective would be:

> By the end of the academic year 2015, 60% of students actively enrolled and participating in the program will understand the basic skills for defusing potentially violent encounters.

There is no way to measure objectively whether someone "understands" the basic skills, even if they perform them. "Understands" can mean different things to different people. More appropriate verb choices for our example might be *demonstrate, list, show,* or *illustrate* "basic skills for defusing potentially violent encounters."

The Condition

The "condition" relates to when the outcome will be observed. The condition is usually expressed in the objective as the date or time by when the outcome can be observed and measured. Some examples of terms and phrases that usually express the condition are "by the end of December 2003," "by June 30, 2004," "after completion of the training program," or "by the end of the class."

Table 14.2. Outcome Verbs for Objectives

1. *Knowledge:*	4. *Analysis:*	7. *Conveying Attitudes:*
define	analyze	acquire
describe	categorize	consider
identify	classify	exemplify
label	differentiate	modify
list	discriminate	plan
match	distinguish	realize
name	infer	reflect
reproduce	select	revise
select	separate	transfer
2. *Comprehension:*	5. *Synthesis:*	8. *Relating to Psychomotor:*
converting	compile	demonstrate
defend	compose	diagnose
describe	conclude	diagram
distinguish	create	empathize
estimate	design	hold
explain	explain	integrate
general	plan	internalize
interpret	propose	listen
paraphrase	revise	massage
predict	summarize	measure
3. *Application:*	synthesize	operate
apply	6. *Evaluating:*	palpate
change	appraise	pass
compute	compare	prepare
discover	conclude	project
illustrate	contrast	record
modify use	describe	visualize
predict	evaluate	write
prepare	explain	
produce	justify	
relate	summarize	
solve	support	

The Criterion

"The criterion" is the third element of the well-written objective. The criterion defines when the outcome is achieved, or how much change will take place. It provides the standard by which the planners can decide if the outcome has been performed "in an appropriate and/or successful manner (McKenzie et al., (2013)." In the earlier example of an objective, the phrase, "60% of students actively enrolled and participating in the program" tells the program planners and the program evaluators the standard for determining if the program is successful. Other examples of a criterion used in an objective are:

". . . 90% of women enrolled in prenatal services . . ."

". . . 80% of enrolled participants 19–24 years old . . ."

The Target

The target population is the fourth element that must be present in the well-written objective. This element tells who will change, such as "60% of *students actively enrolled and participating in the program*. The target population is not "students," but students who are enrolled and participating in the program. Other examples are "HIV+ women of child-bearing age in Pico County," "all infants born to women who are substance abusers," or "All employees of ACE Corporation."

The Hierarchy of Objectives

In order to achieve the goal(s) of a program, it is necessary to address different levels of objectives. Objectives are designed in a hierarchical manner, so that each objective at each level becomes successively more explicit. This means that the achievement of the lower level objectives contributes to the upper level objectives and the goal(s). Deeds (1992) offers a hierarchy of objectives and shows how each level relates to program outcomes, possible evaluation measures, and types of evaluation. The achievement of the lower level objectives (level 1) will contribute the achievement of the higher level objectives (levels 2 and 3) and the goals (McKenzie et al., 2013).

Hierarchy of Objectives and Their Relation to Evaluation

Level 1—Process or Administrative Objectives

The process or administrative objectives are the first level of objectives and include the daily activities and tasks that will lead to the accomplishment of other higher levels of objectives. The process or administrative objectives are the objectives that deal with all program details that shape the program: program resources, the appropriateness of intervention activities, recruitment regimen for the target population, program participation, attendance, feedback from program participants and other stakeholders, data collection methods, etc.

Examples:

- By June 30, 2022, 250 youth aged 12–16 will be recruited to the program.
- Two culturally appropriate brochures will be published for the African American participants' nutrition education needs by December 31, 2022.

Level 2—Impact Objectives

The impact objectives are the second level of objectives. Impact objectives include three different types of objectives: learning objectives, behavioral objectives, and environmental objectives. These objectives are called impact objectives because they reflect the immediate observable effects of the program. They will show changes in awareness, knowledge, attitudes, skills, behaviors, or the environment. These objectives provide the foundation for the impact evaluation.

Learning Objectives

Learning objectives are the educational or learning tools that are needed in order to achieve the planned behavior change. Learning objectives relate to the predisposing, reinforcing, and enabling factors related to change. The learning objectives have their own hierarchy of four different types of learning objectives, moving from the least complex to the most complex. The level of complexity relates to time, effort, and resources necessary to accomplish the learning objectives. The levels for the learning objectives are also related to the learning domains.

1. Awareness objectives (the least complex)
2. Knowledge objectives (relates to the cognitive domain)
3. Attitudes objectives (relates to the affective domain)
4. Skills development or acquisition objectives (relates to the psychomotor domain)

Examine the following learning objectives and determine which of the learning objectives address awareness, knowledge, attitudes, and skill development.

1. ___ By the end of the academic year, 2024, 60% of students actively enrolled and participating in the program will demonstrate the basic skills for defusing potentially violent encounters.

2. ___ After the participants have examined the program brochure on type 2 diabetes; at least 40% will be able to identify all of the risk factors for type 2 diabetes.
3. ___ By the end of the class, 50% of pregnant participants will be able to explain the importance of iron in the diet during pregnancy.
4. ___ At the end of the program, 80% of the adolescent participants will debate their views of the pros and cons of teenage pregnancy.

Answers:

1. skill development
2. awareness
3. knowledge
4. attitude

Behavioral Objectives

Behavioral objectives are based on specific health behaviors that are linked to the identified health problem. Through the problem analysis the planners should have recognized target behaviors that are part of the cause, and effect relationship between the behavior and health issue. These objectives describe the behaviors or actions in which the target population will engage that will resolve the health problem and move toward achieving the program goal. The learning objectives that cover the cognitive, affective, psychomotor domains are written to support the fulfillment of behavioral objectives.

Examples of the behavioral objectives:

▪ One year after the completion of the program, 75% of the program participants who completed the Heart Health course will report having their blood pressure measured weekly during the previous six months.
▪ Six months after the completion of the Diabetes Prevention Program, 70% of the participants completing 90% of the physical activity classes will follow a personal activity regimen for 20 minutes of vigorous activity for each of five days per week.

Environmental Objectives

Environmental objectives address the non-behavioral causes or precursors of or links to health problems that are identified from the needs assessment. The environmental changes may be defined as the physical, social, psychological, or cultural environments.

Example:

▪ By December 30, 2024, 75% of those without health care in Pico County will enroll in a health insurance plan that gives them access to quality health care.
▪ By September 30, 2025, 90% of the low-income communities in Potts City will have access to recreation centers, parks and walking trails.

Level 3—Outcome Objectives

Outcome objectives, also referred to as program objectives, state the ultimate end result or objectives of the program. They are objectives that are "outcome or future-oriented" that deal with changes in quality of life, health status, or social benefits (McKenzie et al., 2013). The outcome objectives are usually written about reductions in risk, mortality, morbidity disability, or quality of life measures. When the outcome objective is accomplished, then the program goal is accomplished.

The success of a program will depend on the selection and specificity of the objectives for solving the problem. All of the levels of objectives should be included in a well-written program plan. This allows for greater opportunities to reach success in a variety of areas that directly relate to the program goal. So be sure to include objectives that are process objectives, impact objectives that include learning objectives, behavioral objectives, and environmental objectives, and outcome objectives in the program plan. In the written program plan, the order for presenting the objectives after the stated goal is usually the outcome objective(s), the impact objectives and then the process objectives. An example of this suggested formatting is presented on page 176.

Most importantly, the objectives and the methods that will be chosen for these objectives must be based on and affect the predisposing, enabling, and reinforcing factors which influence health behaviors and health status. These factors may also be expressed as precursors or risk factors. Every objective must be a SMART objective: SMART stands for specific, measurable, achievable, realistic, and time phased (CDC, 2003).

Program Intervention Methods and Activities

After selecting the goals and objectives, planners must identify the strategy or intervention that leads to the achievement of the goals and objectives. The intervention is the planned method and activity or set of methods and activities that permit the most effective pathway to accomplishing the program goals and objectives, and the most efficient and responsible use of resources. The planning team may be temporarily expanded to include individuals or consultants with special expertise in policy development, educational methods, application of theory, and/or community organization. This allows the team to examine the variety of methods available and then choose the best methods for fulfilling each objective and reaching the program goal.

Methods are considered the general descriptions of how the change within the target population will be accomplished. In health promotion, methods may include community advocacy and development, communications and mass media, educational and instructional methods, counseling and behavior modification, group work, support groups, legislative and regulatory methods, policy development, environmental changes, health status appraisals, etc. In health education the methods are educational methods to change behavior based in learning principles and behavioral theories and models. Various methods will also include activities. The activities are specific events or opportunities used to execute the method and achieve the expected outcome of the objectives. The decision about the most effective and efficient methods and activities is central to the success of the program. Therefore, members of the target population must be consulted and included in the selection of intervention methods and activities. The inclusion of representatives of the target population can ensure that the methods and activities are educationally, culturally and socially relevant and appropriate.

There is abundant literature on various methods and activities that have been used in health promotion programs, and the theories and models upon which they are based. The decision for the best methods and activities must be based on sound rationale. While there is no perfect way to choose a successful method or intervention, the choice has to be more than "chance," "a good feeling" or "sounds good."

Table 14.3 lists some of the more popular and common health education methods used in health education to accomplish program objectives and program goals.

McKenzie and Smeltzer (1997) recommend some major considerations in creating a health promotion intervention. The following questions may serve as criteria for the selection of appropriate methods and activities.

- Are the selected methods based upon appropriate theory?
- Do the program methods and activities fit the goals and objectives of the program?
- Are the necessary resources available to implement the selected intervention, methods and activities?
- Are the intervention methods and activities appropriate for the segmented target audience?
- What types of intervention methods and activities are known to be effective (successful in previous programs and with similar populations) in dealing with the program focus?
- Are the selection of methods and activities informed by evidence based practice and research?
- Would it be better to use an intervention that consists of a single event or one that is made up of multiple events and activities?

The responses o these questions can help to choose appropriate program interventions. Some of the considerations in choosing intervention types and methods are highlighted in the following flow chart for planning program interventions.

Table 14.3.   Listing of Health Education Methods

Getting acquainted/icebreakers	Models
Audio	Music
Audiovisual materials	Newsletters/flyers
Brainstorming	Panels
Case studies	Peer education
Cooperative learning and group work	Personal improvement projects
Computer-assisted instruction	Problem solving
Debates	Puppets
Displays & bulletin boards	Role plays
Educational game	Self-appraisals
Experiments and demonstrations	Simulations
Field trips	Social media
Guest speakers	Storytelling and literary venues
Guided imagery	Theater (using scripts)
Humor	Value clarification
Lecture	Video conferencing
Mass media	Word games and puzzles

Factors to Consider in Creating a Health Education/Promotion Intervention

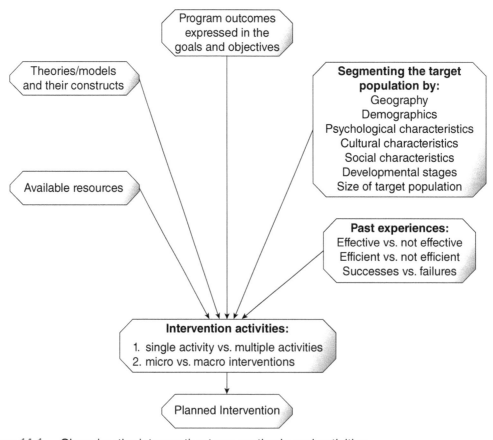

Figure 14.1.   Choosing the intervention type, methods and activities

References

Butler, J. T. 2001. *Principles of Health Education and Health Promotion,* 3rd ed. Belmont, CA: Wadsworth/ Thomas Learning.

Doyle, E., and S. Ward. 2005. *The Process of Community Health Education and Promotion.* Long Grove, IL: Waveland Press, Inc.

Hanson, M. (Ed.). 1997. *Maternal and Child Health Program Design and Development: From the Ground Up; Collaboration and Partnership.* US Department of Health and Human Services, Maternal and Child Health Services.

McKenzie J. F., and J. L. Smeltzer. 1997. *Planning, Implementing and Evaluating Health Promotion Programs: A Primer,* 2nd ed. Boston: Allyn and Bacon.

McKenzie, J. F., B. L. Neiger, and R. Thackeray. 2013. *Planning, Implementing, and Evaluating Health Promotion Programs: A Primer.* Boston: Pearson Education.

Peoples-Sheps MD, A. Farel, and M. M. Rogers. 1996. *Assessment of Health Status Problems.* Washington, DC: Maternal and Child Health Bureau.

Application Opportunity

Activity A

Visit Healthy People 2020 or Healthy People 2030 on the internet and discover additional tools and information that are helpful for program planning, using Healthy People 2020 or Healthy People 2030 objectives.

http://www.healthypeople.gov/2020/tools-and-resources/Program-Planning.

Activity B

Using the low birthweight babies' problem presented in this chapter, the problem statement, the hypothesis, and the mission statement, develop one written goal and appropriate objectives to realize the goal and to address the stated problem. Remember to address the varying levels of objectives.

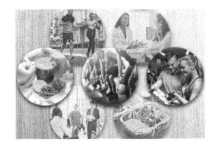

CHAPTER 15
Health Education Process: Planning for Implementation

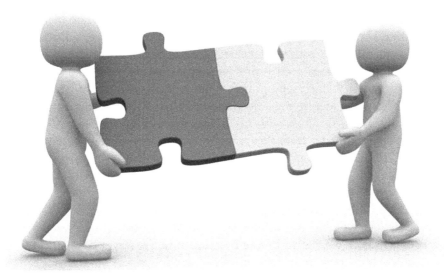

© Liviu Ionut Pantelimon, 2013. Used under license from Shutterstock, Inc.

The planner through the health education process has designed the various components of the program plan that is to be delivered to the target population. After the planning of the program comes the implementation of the program. Generally, implementation means the activation of the program plan. The implementation determines if the planners will be successful in producing the measurable changes, impacts and outcomes identified in the plan's objectives. The details and logistics of implementing a program will differ given the nature and scope of the program, the target population's characteristics, the number and the nature of cooperating organizations involved, the types of personnel to be recruited, hired and trained, needed facilities and equipment, other resources, and constraints. The implementation must be well planned and the roles of all stakeholders, professionals, and organizations clearly delineated. An implementation plan must also provide for appropriate funding and training needs.

Health education specialists must apply a variety of competencies and sub-competencies when fulfilling the responsibility of implementing the program plan. These include, but are not limited to, curriculum development, presentation skills, group facilitation skills, data collection as well as technology utilization (Cottrell et al., 2012).

Implementation requires the health education specialist and the planning team to decide on the appropriate course of action for implementation, to write and execute clear and concise policy statement(s), and implementation plan. The health education specialist will continue to review and examine the role of cultural, social, ethnic, religious, spiritual, and behavioral factors in determining how the program is delivered. The planning team and the health education staff implementing the program will adhere to the code of ethics for health education professionals.

Implementation Considerations

Personnel

Throughout this book, the health education specialist has been the focus for carrying out the health education process. Needless to say, the health education specialist will not carry out all of the duties and responsibilities required for designing, implementing, and evaluating a health education program. The key resource of the health education program will be the people required to carry out the program services. Throughout the needs assessment and the development of the program plan many tasks are revealed for the proper delivery of the program. The health education planner should at first focus on all of the tasks that must be fulfilled in order for the program to go forth rather than trying to think of individuals who might be hired into the program prematurely. Some of the tasks are identifying resources, advertising, marketing, conducting the program, providing support services, services for those with disabilities, translating services with language challenges, evaluating the program, managing data, recordkeeping, budgeting, administrative tasks, etc. After creating the tasks lists, the health education specialist and the planning team can study existing and potential program resources. The planning team will now determine the appropriate positions to fulfill the identified tasks. The planners have internal personnel who are those individuals already working for the agency that is home to the program or they are members of the target population. Sometimes workers in other agency departments will change positions to work in a program after receiving appropriate training. On occasion there may be a need for a worker with certain specialized skills and there is a person in the target population who has that skill. The agency may have student interns from the local university willing to serve in the program or there may be peer educators from the local high school willing to work with other children or youth. The other source of personnel is external or outside of the home planning agency. These may be people outside of the agency who would conduct all or part of the required services. These individuals may only fill in the "gaps" that cannot be filled within the home agency. Others will be hired for a specific position to fulfill tasks. The agency may contract with an outside vendor for a person or persons to provide services to the program. Regardless of the planner's choice, appropriate training for the specific program tasks and services is required in preparation for the program's start.

Fiscal Planning and Budgeting

Program implementation must necessarily include fiscal planning and budgeting. This will assure that appropriate funds and resources are properly matched with fiscal needs and demands. A budgeting process is required to be sure that limited resources are not wasted and that over-expenditures do not occur. The costs of resources that include personnel, materials, equipment, and the program site can make or break the planned program. If the health education specialist is responsible for implementing a program plan that does not have adequate financial resources, then he or she may also be responsible for securing the funds to support the program. This may be done through the health education specialist seeking donations or sponsors, through grant sources, or fund-raising events. How funds are secured for health programming will depend on the agencies' policies and directives. Health education specialist will follow agency protocol in all aspects of implementation. If the health education specialist receives permission to seek donations, be sure that other divisions in the agency are not requesting funds from the same companies or sponsors. Corporate sponsors will usually contribute funding to programs or parts of programs that relate to their own special interests or missions. There is no single way to seek corporate funding. Often contact is made with a potential donor with a letter, a face-to-face meeting or a telephone call. Again, be certain that the funds that they will donate can be accepted by the planner and the agency. The health professional must not overwhelm a donor with excessive requests.

Grant funding is a very common way to secure funds. There are a great number of federal, state, and local government agencies that offer money for health programs. Funding is also offered for health programs by many voluntary agencies (i.e., American Heart Association, the American Cancer Society, etc.), foundations, and professional organizations. There are even private individuals who offer funds to support health programming in which they are interested. It is strongly suggested that health education specialists spend time on the internet and identify the many agencies that would provide grant funding for a specific health program. In most cases grant funding begins with an application completed by the appropriate agency official and submitted to the funding organization. Most of these organizations will request a program proposal. Grant proposal writing has much in common with the process of developing a program plan. The program plan can inform the grant writing. The main difference in the two is that the grant proposal is usually a strongly competitive process. The funding of the program plan will depend on how well the planner can write the proposal so that it will be chosen for funds above all other proposals submitted to the funding organization. Doyle and Ward (1997, p. 176) share tips for successful grant proposals.

The successful grant proposal:

- Perfectly adheres to the funder's requirements.
- Will be based on an innovative idea. Even if it is an old idea put in a new and innovative package.
- Will advance the practice of health education and/or community health.
- Will fill a critical gap in knowledge and/or care.
- Will be driven by sound evidence, theory, and research.
- Works toward a long-term goal.
- Includes a thoughtful and up-to-date literature review.
- Is well-written.
- Provides evidence of feasibility.
- Demonstrates an appropriate choice of methods.
- Is well-focused.
- Has a well-thought out evaluation plan.

Pilot-Testing, Phasing in, and Total Implementation

Health education specialists will plan the implementation of a program based on available resources and the setting for which the program is intended. However, it is important to consider three critical factors that contribute to the success of health program plans. Health promotion programs work well when the implementation addresses the following:

1. The recipients are recognized, respected, and treated as contributors throughout the planning, implementation, and evaluation of the program.
2. Those responsible for delivering the program are qualified and competent.
3. There is responsible evaluation and reporting of the program's impacts and outcomes.

Three major ways of implementing a program are suggested by Parkinson et al., (1982): pilot testing, phasing-in, and initiating the total program.

Pilot-Testing

Pilot testing (piloting or field testing) a program permits the health education specialist and staff to implement the program on a small scale with a small number of the target population. Pilot testing allows the planners to have close control of the program. It enables the planners to identify and solve any problems that may exist before the program is offered to a larger number of the target population. Ideally the pilot testing should occur with people who are like the target population and in a similar setting. Planners will want to be sure that:

1. staff selection and training are adequate and appropriate.
2. planned methods and activities work.
3. program is marketed appropriately.
4. facilities are appropriate.
5. program timelines, schedules, and logistics are worked out.
6. program participants are given the opportunity to evaluate the program.

The evaluation of the program by the participants is part of process evaluation or formative evaluation. The participants are able to evaluate program content, methods and activities, practitioner or instructor effectiveness, facilities and space, accommodations, etc. As a result of the process feedback, planners will make changes in the program. If many changes are made, it may be necessary to pilot test the program again.

Phasing In

When there is a very large target population, pilot testing should be followed by the phasing in of the program rather than implementing the full program. Phasing in the program allows the planner to have greater control over the program. It helps to prevent planners and program staff from being overwhelmed. Phasing in the program can be done by setting up various stages by using the following techniques to control the number of participants coming into the program:

1. limiting the number of participants from the target group entering the program at one time; set up intervals for admissions.
2. choice of location or setting; time the start of programs in different settings, so they do not all begin at once.
3. addressing a particular skill level of the participants; instead of bringing all residents in a setting into the program. For a community project that serves everyone in a given location, it may be more manageable to begin with parents first, then adolescents and then the children ten and younger.
4. offering particular aspects of the program activities. Instead of offering the whole program to a population, some participants could begin with one program feature while others begin a different program feature. Eventually all participants will participate in all offerings, but not all at one time.

Example:

If Pico County Health Department wanted to phase in their planned HIV Prevention Program for women of childbearing age, the planners might do the following things to phase in the program.

1. Limiting the number of participants from the target group.
   The implementation of the program will be focused on adolescents and young adults. With each new quarter of the year, services for a new age group will be added.
2. Choice of location or setting.
   The program is implemented only in the northwest part of the county for the first four months. The next four months of the program services will be offered in the northwest part of the county and in the southeast part of the county. Every four months, a new part of the county is added until the total county is receiving the program services.
3. Addressing a particular skill level of the participants.
   If the program included activities for increasing physical activity levels, the planners might start with beginning exercisers. Then in three months add services for intermediate exercisers. Finally, services would be added for advanced exercisers.
4. Offering particular aspects of the program activities.
   Planners may decide to begin program services with classes in stress management, and then add assertiveness training.

Total Implementation

Seldom would total implementation be appropriate without the pilot testing and phasing in processes. Pilot testing and phasing in will lead to necessary revisions in the program and the resolution of identified problems in the program's implementation. Total implementation can only benefit significantly from the pilot-testing and the phasing in. However, in some instances, only total implementation is possible. Programs that are planned or implemented around a single event, such as a lecture, screening event, or a one day health fair are exceptions; the health education specialist would offer the total program all at once for these types of events.

Other Concerns

Informed Consent

The well-being of the program participants is of primary concern. Every participant must be fully informed about the benefits and the risks of participating in the program. Informed consent from the participant is a requirement for any individual participating in any health promotion program. McKenzie et al., (2013) suggest that program facilitators prepare participants for obtaining informed consent by doing the following:

1. Explain the nature and purpose of the program.
2. Inform program participants of any inherent risks or dangers associated with participation and any possible discomfort they may experience.
3. Explain the expected benefits of participation.
4. Inform participants of alternative programs or procedures that will accomplish the same thing.
5. Indicate to the participants that they are free to discontinue participation at any time.

Health education specialists must know that the participant's signing of the informed consent documents is not a release of liability or waiver of liability. If the health education specialist or any program staff person is negligent they can be found liable.

Policies and Procedures

The health education specialist and the program staff will address how the program moves toward the fulfillment of its goals and objectives through specific written policies and procedures. These will need regular review and updating in order to be relevant for the target population(s) and the program personnel delivering the services. Careful thought and preparation should be involved in policy development. Who will have the responsibility for developing policies and procedures? Who will administer the policies? Who in the agency will approve and oversee the policies and procedures?

Timeline

A tentative timetable can be very helpful in keeping the health education specialist and the program staff on task for program implementation. Such a timetable can be useful for all of the planning and implementation processes. An example of a planning and implementation timetable is included on the next page. Every responsibility of the planners and the program staff must be scheduled and that schedule must guide the development and implementation of the program. Those who are responsible for the planning and implementation might prefer a more detailed schedule or calendar and for a longer period of time, if required.

Reporting

Planners will need to document and report the ongoing progress of the program to the target population, other stakeholders, administrators, and the community. The documentation and reporting is vitally important (1) for keeping the current participants motivated; (2) for recruiting new participants; (3) for public relations and for keeping the community involved; (4) for accountability.

Sample Timeline for Planning, Implementation, and Evaluation

Programming Tasks Year 1	Responsible Personnel	JAN	FEB	MAR	APR	MAY	JUN	JUL	AUG	SEP	OCT	NOV	DEC
Assemble the planning committee.	Project Director	X											
Conduct the needs assessment.	Planning Committee		X	X									
Develop hypothesis, goals, and objectives.	Planning Committee				X	X							
Review policies and rules.	Planning Committee				X	X							
Design intervention/methods/activities.	Project Staff						X	X					
Assemble resources.	Project Manager						X	X					
Market the program.	Project Staff & Planning Committee									X	X		
Recruit program participants.	Project Staff									X	X		
Pilot test program.	Nurses and Health Educators											X	X
Process evaluation.	Project evaluator and staff											X	X

Programming Tasks Year 2	Responsible Personnel	JAN	FEB	MAR	APR	MAY	JUN	JUL	AUG	SEP	OCT	NOV	DEC
Review and revise the program.	Project Staff	X	X										
Market the program.	Project staff & Planning Committee				X	X							
Recruit program participants.	Project staff				X	X							
Phase in Part 1.	Nurses & Health Educators						X	X					
Phase in Part 2.	Nurses & Health Educators								X	X			
Total implementation.	Nurses & Health Educators										X	X	
Impact evaluation.	Project staff										X	X	
Prepare evaluation report.	Project Evaluator											X	
Distribute report.	Project Director												X

Cultural Competence

As mentioned in other places in this text, the health education specialists are urged to include responsible representatives of the target population and other stakeholders who are respected and trusted by the community. They must be involved throughout the planning, implementation, and evaluation stages of the program. To accomplish this and to be successful with the program, cultural competence is required. Cultural competence is based on the principle that all individuals are to be treated equally, respectfully, and are to receive the best and appropriate care regardless of race, ethnicity, culture, religion, or creed. The health education specialist, the planning team, and the program staff must demonstrate cultural competency throughout the planning, implementation, and evaluation of the program. It may be the responsibility of the health education specialist to train the program staff in cultural competence. It is important that the staff treat all persons, even their fellow workers with respect, honoring each person for who he or she is and what they bring to the program. All persons should receive the same respect and quality of service and communication in the program operations. This is not a matter of race or color because culture is so much more than that. The goals must be offering quality health care to all people and overcoming barriers to the access to quality health services.

The Office of Minority Health and Health Equity, US Department of Health and Human Services offers this reminder about the importance of cultural competence in health professionals:

> . . . It's the way patients and doctors can come together and talk about health concerns without cultural differences hindering the conversation, but enhancing it. Quite simply, health care services that are respectful of and responsive to the health beliefs, practices and cultural and linguistic needs of diverse patients can help bring about positive health outcomes. (OMH, 2013)

The implementation plan must include a marketing plan to reach the target population with an outreach system and messaging that is respectful, ethical and addresses the cultural sensitivities of the target population. The program offered must be of the highest quality given the program resources to achieve program goals and objectives.

References

Butler, J. T. 2001. *Principles of Health Education and Health Promotion,* 3rd ed. Belmont, CA: Wadsworth/ Thomas Learning.

Doyle, E., and S. Ward. 2005. *The Process of Community Health Education and Promotion.* Long Grove, IL: Waveland Press, Inc.

Huff, R. M., and M. V. Kline. 1999. *Promoting Health in Multicultural Populations, a Handbook for Practitioners.* Thousand Oaks: Sage Publications.

McKenzie, J. F., B. L. Neiger, and R. Thackeray. 2013. *Planning, Implementing, and Evaluating Health Promotion Programs: A Primer.* Boston: Pearson Education.

Office of Minority Health. 2013. *What is Cultural Competency?* Retrieved on June 12, 2013 at http://www .minorityhealth.hhs.gov/templates/browse.aspx?lvl=2&lvlid=11.

Simons-Morton, B. G., W. H. Greene, and N. H. Gottlieb. 1995. *Introduction to Health Education and Health Promotion.* Prospect Heights, IL: Waveland.

Specter, R. 2009. *Cultural Diversity in Health and Illness.* Upper Saddle River, NJ: Pearson/Prentice Hall.

Application Opportunity

A Case Study

Juanita is a health educator who has worked with the King Mountain community for the past year addressing the increased incidence of HIV infection among women of childbearing ages. The King Mountain community is predominantly Non–Hispanic Caucasian (40%), Hispanic (36%) and African American (23%), and quite diverse economically. The community has a long history in community activism. It is also a community with a strong spiritual tradition among African Americans and Hispanics. Juanita and her planning committee have designed a HIV prevention program for women of childbearing ages 18–25 years old. They are having difficulty deciding where to implement the program. The community representatives want the program offered through the neighborhood churches. The professional health representatives are uncomfortable with this suggestion, because they do not think that religious institutions have a role in health matters.

1. If you were Juanita, what would you do to resolve this issue?

2. Is the recommendation of the community representatives realistic and relevant? Why or why not?

3. Is the position of the professional health representatives a real concern? Why or why not?

4. What successful models for a partnership between the health department and the faith community already exist in your community and in other communities?

Case Study Resources

Eng, E., J. Hatch, A. Callan. 1985. "Institutionalizing social support through the church and into the community." *Health Education Quarterly* 12 (1): 81–92. DOI: 10.1177/109019818501200107

Sutton, M. Y., and C. P. Parks. 2013. "HIV/AIDS Prevention, Faith, and Spirituality among Black/ African American and Latino Communities in the United States: Strengthening Scientific Faith-Based Efforts to Shift the Course of the Epidemic and Reduce HIV-Related Health Disparities." *Journal of Religion & Health* 52 (2): 514–30. DOI: 10.1007/s10943-011-9499-z

The Center for Faith-based and Neighborhood Partnerships http://www.hhs.gov/partnerships/

National Heart, Lung, and Blood Institute Faith—Based Tool Kit http://www.nhlbi.nih.gov/ educational/hearttruth/materials/faith-based-toolkit.htm

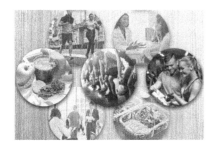

CHAPTER 16
Health Education Process: Planning for Program Evaluation

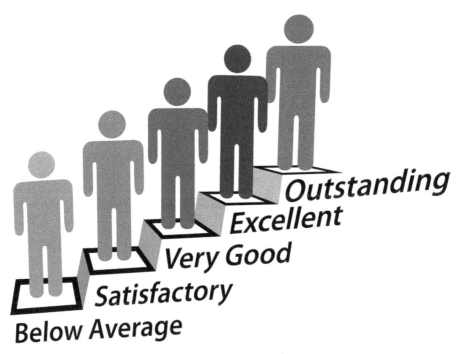

©Photographer/Shutterstock.com

Program evaluation is crucial to health education and health promotion programming and serves many purposes. A plan for program evaluation is developed as the goals, objectives, and methods are developed for the program plan. If the objectives for changed behavior and health status are written correctly they will yield the measures needed to evaluate the program. Without well-written and SMART objectives there is no reliable program evaluation.

Evaluation unfortunately is often misunderstood. Butler (2001) identifies some of the reasons why evaluation is misunderstood. Students often view evaluation as a test for which they must cram to get a good grade. Health education specialists sometimes see evaluation as the laborious task of filling out forms that only result in meetings with supervisors to discuss their deficiencies. Supervisors, planners, and teachers may see evaluation as a way of enforcing discipline on employees and students. Evaluation is none of these. Program evaluation is none of these things.

Evaluation Purpose

Purpose

In most planning models for health promotion, evaluation is mentioned last. However, evaluation actually occurs in all phases of program-planning. It occurs at the beginning, as well as at the end, and anywhere in-between, if required. Evaluation is basically the comparison of an object or objective of interest against a standard of acceptability. "Standards of acceptability are the minimum levels of performance, effectiveness, or benefits used to judge value" (McKenzie et al., 2013). The more common standards of acceptability may include, but are not limited to, comparison or control groups, norms, values, and mandates (policies, statutes, and laws) that are supported by research, evaluations of previous programs, or implementation protocols.

The overall purpose of evaluation is not to prove or disprove anything, but it is to assess and improve the health program quality (Creswell and Newman, 1993). McKenzie et al., (2013) add that evaluation also determines program effectiveness. Evaluation should be a nonthreatening, positive force for health promotion that may have these added benefits: offer knowledge, attitudes, and practices related to health, serve as a foundation for constructing objectives for instruction; determine the value of learning experiences and teaching strategies; assess attainment of desired outcomes, goals, and objectives; assess accomplishments of the program; identify limitations or weaknesses of the program; assess the value of learning aids and materials and the ways in which they have been used; determine the level of achievement for each individual student/client, as well as for the group; and justify the program and its expenditures (Butler, 2001).

Elder et al., (1994) describes evaluation as the systematic process of collecting and analyzing reliable and valid information at various points and processes in the program in order to improve program effectiveness, reduce costs and to contribute to future planning efforts. Program evaluation must always emphasize reliable, valid and systematic information and does not really differ in substance from "real" research. However, through its orientation toward quality enhancement, cost effectiveness, and planning, program evaluation may take on a much different tone than its epidemiological or clinical trial counterparts (Elder et al., 1994). Thus evaluation must yield accurate information to determine the process, impact and outcome of health education and health promotion programs and health services. It also enables planners to make decisions based on accurate information and not on speculation.

Who Conducts the Evaluation?

Planners will have to determine who conducts the evaluation. Evaluators must avoid conflict of interest and be as objective as possible. The evaluator may be someone associated with the program or someone who is external to the program. The internal evaluator is someone who has the advantage of being closer to the program staff and activities, so the collection of relevant information is easier. The internal evaluator is less expensive usually than hiring additional staff to conduct the evaluation. The disadvantage of using the internal evaluator is the possibility of evaluator bias. Certainly someone involved in the program has an investment in its outcome.

The external evaluator is usually more objective, but also more expensive than the internal evaluator. The external evaluator of course has less experience with the program and should provide unbiased evaluation results. The program planners may find it helpful to employ consultants with evaluation expertise to develop the evaluation plan.

Writing Measurable Objectives for Program Evaluation

As stated earlier, goals are general statements about the proposed changes in health status and/or quality of life for a target or priority population. They give the future big picture of what the program plan will accomplish for the population. Goals provide a sense of where the planners and the population want to go, but they give us no specific steps on how to reach the destination.

Objectives are the measurable statements that will lead to the accomplishment of the program goals. Earlier the reader was instructed on how to write effective and measurable objectives. There are a variety of instructions from credible sources on how to write measurable objectives. The key is that the well-written objective is a clear directive on how to reach a program goal. Objectives are process objectives, impact objectives or outcome objectives. These then align themselves with the categories of evaluation in one framework: process evaluation, impact evaluation, and outcome evaluation (Green & Kreuter, 1991). The program planners must be sure to include the key elements in every objective: the outcome to be achieved (what will change); the condition under which the outcome will be observed (when will the change occur); the criterion for deciding whether the outcome has been achieved (how much change is proposed); and the priority population or the target population (who will change). The objective that is well-written serves to guide the program staff on the methods and activities that must be implemented effectively, what data must be collected and measured to determine if the objective has accomplished what was originally planned.

Evaluation Terminology

The health educator or program evaluator will use the evaluation framework that aligns with the categories of the objectives to provide guidance in planning the evaluation. There are generally two sets of terminology and frameworks used by authors addressing levels or types of evaluation. Some professionals use the terms process, impact, and outcome evaluations, while others use the terms diagnostic, formative, and summative evaluations.

The first framework discussed here has three levels of evaluation (Green and Kreuter, 1991) and asks different questions about the program or activity, addresses different aspects of the program or its effects, and deals with different indicators. Process evaluation examines how well the program or activity being implemented relates to the actual program plan. Impact evaluation determines the changes that occur in the target population's knowledge, attitudes, beliefs, values, skills, behaviors, and practices as the result of the program or intervention. Impact evaluation also measures changes in policies, programs and resources at the organizational level. At the organizational or governmental levels, impact evaluation may show changes in policies, plans, legislation and funding related to given issues. Outcome evaluation identifies the improvements in health or social factors as the result of the intervention. Outcome evaluation examines the health status of the target population, morbidity rates that are at issue, and mortality rates that are at issue. Figure 16.1 illustrates process, impact, and outcome evaluation and the types of data collected and measured for each. The needs assessment is considered an important part of the evaluation process in this framework and is included in the diagram. The needs assessment provides much of the baseline data.

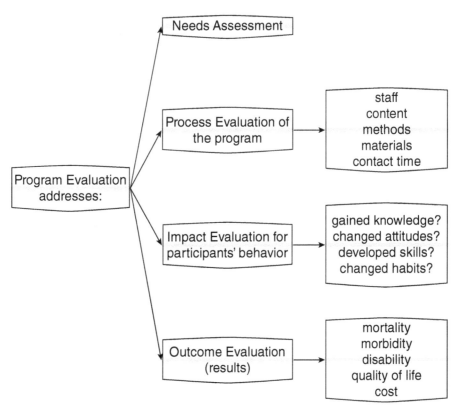

Figure 16.1.   Process, impact, outcome, and related data measurements

The second framework includes the terms diagnostic, formative and summative evaluation. Diagnostic evaluation is the needs assessment. It commonly applies to individuals and groups to determine their needs for knowledge, attitude change, behavior change, or skill development. Formative evaluation begins when the program is being formed and continues throughout the program implementation to identify needed adjustments in the program. Formative evaluation is closely aligned with process evaluation. After the program is completed, the summative evaluation is implemented to examine all measurements and data that leads to judgments about the impact and outcomes of the program and to determine if the program should continue or to identify needed modifications prior to the program's next operation. The second framework for evaluation is presented in Figure 16.2 and indicates the measurements and data for this evaluation framework.

The Evaluation Plan

Despite the great value that evaluation provides for the program staff, participants, stakeholders, community and funding agencies, there may be instances when it is not included in the program or it is poorly executed. This observation underscores the importance of health educators and health promoters being qualified to design, plan and execute credible program evaluation. The responsibilities and competencies of the health education specialist includes a specific responsibility and competencies for conducting evaluation and research related to health education. The reader is referred to Area of Responsibility IV to examine the competencies required of the certified health education specialist for planning program evaluation.

The health educator must not only plan the health education/health promotion program, but he/she must be able to plan the program's evaluation. Doyle and Ward (2005) suggest that the evaluation plan for a health education program must contain, but are not limited to, the following components:

1. Include target population, stakeholders and program planners in the evaluation planning
2. Evaluation objectives that are linked to the program objectives and reflects how the program objectives will be measured

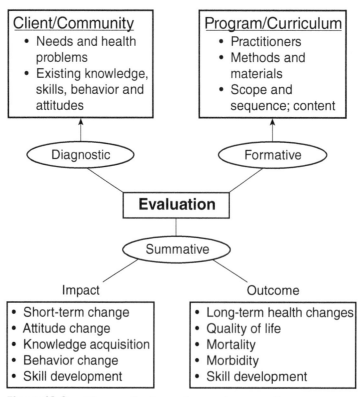

Figure 16.2. Diagnostic, formative and summative components of evaluation

3. A study design that clearly identifies the selected population(s), the types of evaluation and methods to be conducted for collecting data for the evaluation. Will your data be collected through interviews, focus groups, clinical tests, or pre- and post-test? Will you collect quantitative and/or qualitative data? What will be the protocols for the collection of the data?
4. Creating a timeline for all evaluation activities that is aligned with the program planning and implementation timelines
5. Establishing a budget for the evaluation that identifies the specific costs for evaluation (Includes personnel, supplies, professional services, consultants, etc.)
6. Selecting, adjusting or designing the instruments to be used for data collection that are valid and reliable
7. Establishing and implementing plans for data analyses
8. Determining the report style and its audience.

Presented here is an example of a program being developed by health education specialist Laura. She has developed the program's mission statement, program goal and objectives. Can you determine what kind of evaluation would be used for each objective (process, impact, or outcome or diagnostic, formative or summative)? What data is needed to measure the objective? How will you collect the data that is needed to measure the objectives?

In the Pico County Health Department, Laura is responsible for designing a series of HIV/AID Prevention workshops for women of childbearing age. She is working on the orientation workshop design and implementation and "Method 1: Health Appraisal." What would her evaluation plan include for this workshop and how will it fit in the overall evaluation plan that she should have for this program? The program's mission statement, goals, objectives, and some methods are offered here.

The Pico County Women's HIV Prevention Program

Mission Statement

The mission of the Pico County Women's HIV Prevention Program is to provide a range of services that will reduce the HIV infection rate among women of child-bearing age. It is expected that this program will result in the reduction of morbidity and mortality among women and children who are at risk, by preventing HIV infection.

Goal

To reduce the incidence of HIV infection among women of child-bearing age in Pico County.

Objectives

Outcome objective

By the end of the year 2025, there will be a 20% reduction in the incidence of HIV infection among the women of childbearing age in Pico County.

Impact objectives:

A. *Behavioral objectives*
   1. By the end of the program, 60% of the women abusing drugs will terminate their drug abuse behavior.
   2. By the end of the program, 60% of the program participants who have been involved in risky sexual behavior will terminate that behavior.
B. *Environmental objectives*
   1. By the end of the program's first year, 50% of the churches in target communities will participate in recruiting women who are high risk for HIV infection, to the program through trained peer advisors in the churches.

2. By the end of the program's first year, 50% of the churches in the target communities will offer a program of support services to program participants in their communities, through trained peer advisors in the churches.

C. *Learning objectives*

1. Awareness Level

   At the end of the program orientation session, 85% of the women participating in the session will be able to identify their own risks for HIV infection.

2. Knowledge Level

   By October 31, 2022, 75% of the participants will explain how HIV is transmitted.

3. Attitude Level

   By the third session, the program participants will express their views on how women can best protect themselves from HIV infection.

4. Skill Development/Acquisition Level

   By the completion of the Pico County Women's HIV Prevention Program, 75% of the participants will be able to demonstrate at least two stress management methods taught to them, that they use to reduce stress in their lives.

Process objectives

1. By August 30, 2022, 250 women of child-bearing age who are at risk for HIV infection will participate in the Pico County Women's HIV Prevention Program.
2. By August 30, 2022, all learning materials and outreach materials will be culturally competent in design and content.

Intervention strategy (strategies) to meet these objectives

Method 1: Health status appraisal

Activity 1A: Each participant attends the Orientation Session. Each participant completes the health appraisal form during the program participants' orientation session. The discussion leader introduces each participant to the concepts of risk factors and protective factors and how they impact their health status. Each participant determines her own health risk factors for HIV.

Method 2: Counseling

Activity 2A: Each participant is assigned to a personal counselor who provides support and guidance as each participant develops a plan for behavior change, implements her plan, monitors and evaluates the changes and outcomes. Participant must meet with and work with her counselor at least once per week.

Method 3: Group work

Activity 3A: Each program participant is assigned to a support group of approximately 10 women participating in the program. The group meets once every two weeks to gain new information, learn and practice new skills that promote health, and to pro-vide support and accountability.

Reporting the Evaluation Results

The program evaluator must generate a final report that includes the data analyses, interpretation, and results to the stakeholders. Usually the number and types of reports are decided at the beginning of the evaluation based on the needs of the stakeholders. The evaluation reports must be timely to achieve important program improvements. The program evaluator must write the report and/or deliver the report orally so that it is communicated to all audiences.

Table 16.1.   Format for an Evaluation Report

Abstract/executive summary	Overview of the program and evaluation. General results, conclusions, and recommendations.
Introduction	Purpose of the evaluation. Program and participant description (including staff, materials, activities, procedures, etc.). Goals and objectives. Evaluation questions.
Methods/procedures	Design of the evaluation. Target population. Instrument Sampling procedures. Data collection procedures. Pilot study results. Validity and reliability. Limitations. Data analyses procedures.
Results	Description of findings from data analyses. Answers to evaluation questions. Addresses any special concerns. Explanation of findings. Charts and graphs of findings.
Conclusions/ recommendations	Interpretation of results. Conclusions about program effectiveness. Program recommendations. Determining if additional information is needed.

The format of the evaluation report is similar to that used for research reports. McKenzie et al., (2013) offer a description of the evaluation report, as summarized in Table 16.1.

References

Butler, J. T. 2001. *Principles of Health Education and Health Promotion*, 3rd ed. Belmont, CA: Wadsworth/ Thomas Learning.

Centers for Disease Control and Prevention. 1999. *Evaluation Steps*. Retrieved on June 11, 2013 at http://www. cdc.gov/eval/steps/index.htm.

Centers for Disease Control and Prevention. 1999. "Framework for Program Evaluation in Public Health." *MMWR* 48 (No. RR-11): 1–40.

Creswell, Jr., W. H. and I. M. Newman. 1993. *School Health Practice (10th edition)*. St. Louis: Times Mirror/ Mosby.

Doyle, E., and S. Ward. 2005. *The Process of Community Health Education and Promotion*. Long Grove, IL: Waveland Press, Inc.

Elder, J. P., S. A. McGraw, and E. J. Stone, et al. 1994. "Catch-Process Evaluation of Environmental-Factors and Programs." *Health Education Quarterly* Supplement: 2. S107–S127.

Giger, J. N., and R. E. Davidhizar. 1995. *Transcultural Nursing Assessment and Intervention*, 2nd ed. St. Louis: Mosby-Year Book.

Green, L. W., and M. W. Kreuter. 1999. *Health Promotion Planning: An Educational and Ecological Approach*. MountainView, CA: Mayfield.

McKenzie, J. F., B. L. Neiger, and R. Thackeray. 2013. *Planning, Implementing, and Evaluating Health Promotion Programs: A Primer*. Boston: Pearson Education.

Peoples-Sheps MD, A. Farel, and M. M. Rogers. 1996. *Assessment of Health Status Problems*. Washington, DC: Maternal and Child Health Bureau.

Simons-Morton, B. G., W. H. Greene, and N. H. Gottlieb. 1995. *Introduction to Health Education and Health Promotion*. Prospect Heights, IL: Waveland.

Application Opportunity

Given what you have learned about program evaluation, develop a written evaluation plan for the Pico County Women's HIV Prevention Program based on the program's mission statement, goals, objectives, methods and activities. You may use either of the evaluation frameworks presented in this chapter for guidance in developing your evaluation plan.

The response will be a sample of an evaluation plan based on the case study in chapter 16, pages 191–192. The evaluation objectives in the sample evaluation plan will address the following:

- at least one process objective
- two learning objectives
- two behavioral and/or environmental objectives
- the outcome objective

In each evaluation objective you will describe:

- at least one evaluation measure for each objective
- who is being evaluated
- who would conduct the evaluation
- when the evaluation occurs

CPSIA information can be obtained
at www.ICGtesting.com
Printed in the USA
LVHW010326150120
643534LV00003B/9